Electrolytes, Body Fluids
and Acid Base Balance

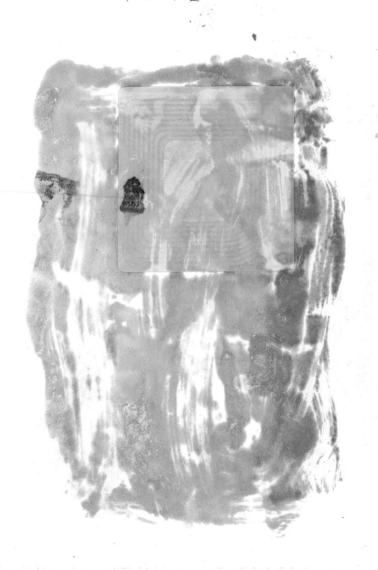

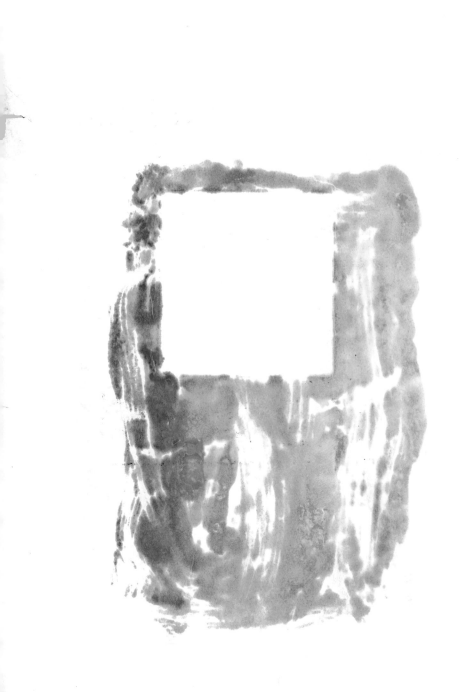

Electrolytes, Body Fluids and Acid Base Balance

R. Eccles BSc, PhD, DSc,

Reader in Physiology,
University of Wales College of Cardiff,
Cardiff

Edward Arnold
A division of Hodder & Stoughton
LONDON BOSTON MELBOURNE AUCKLAND

© 1993 R. ECCLES

First published in Great Britain 1993

Distributed in the Americas by Little, Brown and Company
34 Beacon Street, Boston, MA 02108

British Library Cataloguing in Publication Data

Eccles, Ronald
  Electrolytes, Body Fluids and Acid-base
  Balance
  I. Title
  612.3

  ISBN 0–340–56754–6

Whilst the advice and information in this book is believed to be true and
accurate at the date of going to press, neither the author nor the publisher
can accept any legal responsibility or liability for any errors or omissions
that may be made. In particular (but without limiting the generality of the
preceding disclaimer) every effort has been made to check drug dosages;
however, it is still possible that errors have been missed. Furthermore,
dosage schedules are constantly being revised and new side effects
recognised. For these reasons the reader is strongly urged to consult the
drug companies' printed instructions before administering any of the drugs
recommended in this book.

Typeset in 10/11 Times by Wearset, Boldon, Tyne and Wear.
Printed in Great Britain for Edward Arnold, a division of Hodder and
Stoughton Limited, Mill Road, Dunton Green, Sevenoaks, Kent
TN13 2YA by St. Edmundsbury Press Ltd, and bound by
Hunter and Foulis Ltd, Edinburgh.

Contents

Preface

This book is aimed at the postgraduate medical student preparing for examinations which require an understanding of electrolytes and acid-base metabolism. The topics are presented in a concise way to aid revision but with suffcient explanation of the basic physiology to ensure a proper grasp of the clinical problems related to disturbances of normal function. The book attempts to bridge the gap between the basic sciences and clinical practice and therefore will also be of use to medical students who wish to obtain a more clinical approach to their basic science course in physiology.

Much of the material in the book has been developed from lectures in applied physiology given to surgeons preparing for primary Fellow of the Royal College of Surgeons (FRCS) and Arab Board examinations. In discussions with these students I found that electrolytes and acid-base balance were the subjects they had most difficulty in understanding. The difficulty in understanding this area often arose from the fact that these subjects received very little attention during the preclinical years. This is why the first chapters in this book revise the basic preclinical physiology to give a sound foundation for the clinical disturbances discussed in later chapters.

This book does not attempt to discuss the latest research but aims to present the topics in a straightforward and understandable form. Since it attempts to summarise the topics, detailed literature references have not been provided and controversial areas have not been dealt with in detail.

This book would not have been written without the help and encouragement of many persons and in particular I need to thank my family for their support in this project and the many trainee surgeons and physicians whose comments and questions during lectures have helped to create what I hope will be a useful book to guide them in their studies.

Ronald Eccles
1993

Abbreviations

ADH	anti-diuretic hormone
ANP	atrial natriuretic peptide
Cl^-	chloride
Ca^{++}	calcium
Ccr	creatinine clearance
CO_2	carbon dioxide
ECF	extracellular fluid
GFR	glomerular filtration rate
HCO_3^-	bicarbonate
H^+	hydrogen
ICF	intracellular fluid
Int F	interstitial fluid
GIT	gastrointestinal
K^+	potassium
meq	milliequivalent
Mg^{++}	magnesium
mmol	millimole
mosmol	milliosmole
O_2	oxygen
P	partial pressure of gas
PAH	para amino hippuric acid
Pcr	plasma concentration of creatinine
PTH	parathyroid hormone
SIADH	syndrome of inappropriate ADH
[ ]	square brackets indicate concentration, e.g. $[Na^+]$

1   Electrolytes and body fluids

The diagnosis and treatment of electrolyte disorders is a skill learned by experience and practice at the bedside but like all clinical skills it is dependent on a proper understanding of the basic sciences. Definition of an equivalent or osmole may appear to be of only academic interest when confronted with a sick patient, but there is a core of basic science knowledge which is essential for the proper understanding and treatment of electrolyte disorders. As with all basic science it is better to begin at the beginning and in this case that means the beginning of life.

Animal life is believed to have originated in the sea and our ancestors, as primitive unicellular organisms, would have been surrounded by sea water which had a composition not too remote from the extracellular fluid surrounding the cells of the human body today. If this speculation seems too remote from life today it is a sobering thought to consider that we all started life as a unicellular fertilised ovum immersed in the secretions of the uterus and in this condition our lifestyle closely resembles that of our distant ancestors.

The movement of life from the sea to land has only been achieved by enclosing a fluid environment similar to sea water and carrying it around on land. In this respect we are still living in a watery environment as every single living cell in the body is surrounded by extracellular fluid whose composition is closely regulated by the organ systems.

The surface of the body is covered by a layer of dead cells forming the skin which acts as an impermeable envelope around the body fluids and restricts water loss due to evaporation. We are still very dependent on ready access to water for our survival and man cannot survive for more than a couple of days without a source of fresh water. Dehydration is still a major cause of loss of human life, not due to lack of water but due to excessive loss of water associated with vomiting and diarrhoea due to gastro-intestinal infection. Millions of lives are lost each year in developing countries from disorders of fluid and electrolyte balance which are readily treatable with fluid and electrolyte therapy.

A proper understanding of the control of fluid and electrolyte balance is essential for the clinician and this can only be achieved by considering the extracellular fluid as a watery environment whose composition is critical to the function of every organ, tissue and cell in the body.

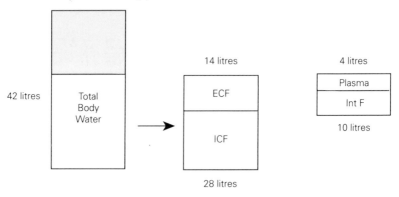

Fig. 1.1   Body fluid compartments. Total body water is divided into extracellular fluid (ECF) and intracellular fluid (ICF) compartments. The ECF can be further divided into an intravascular compartment (plasma) and interstitial fluid (Int F). Na^+ is the major cation of extracellular fluid and K^+ the major cation of intracellular fluid.

Body water and fluid compartments

Water is the main constituent of the body and total body water varies with age and sex and ranges from 45–60% of body weight or 40–45 litres of water. Normal males have around 60% of body weight as water and females 52% of body weight. The lower percentage of water in the female is due to the higher fat content of the body.

Body water can be divided into two compartments: intracellular fluid (ICF) as the major compartment comprising two thirds of body water and extracellular fluid (ECF) making up the remaining one third of body water. The body fluid compartments are illustrated in Fig. 1.1. Of the total body water of around 42 litres, plasma only comprises four litres. Despite the relatively small volume of plasma this is a vital fluid as the composition of plasma influences the composition of the extracellular fluid around all the cells of the body. Plasma is circulated around the body via the cardiovascular system and changes in the composition of plasma affect all cells.

Electrolytes

An electrolyte is defined as a compound which dissociates into ions in solution. Electrolytes are important regulators of nervous and metabolic activity and the concentration gradients for electrolytes between the intracellular and extracellular compartments are utilised to move ions and control cellular activity.

Electrolytes dissociate in solution to form a positively charged cation and a negatively charged anion. The numbers of cations and anions in any solution must always balance. A solution of sodium chloride NaCl con-

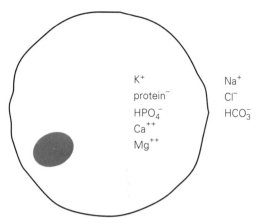

Fig. 1.2 Electrolytes. There are major differences in the concentrations of electrolytes in the intracellular and extracellular compartments. K^+ is the dominant cation in the intracellular compartment and Na^+ in the extracellular compartment.

tains equal numbers of Na^+ cations and Cl^- anions and some undissociated NaCl.

The body fluids contain a complex mixture of cations and anions together with solutes such as glucose and urea. Despite the complexity of the solution the electrical charges on the cations and anions always balance.

The major cations found in body fluids are Na^+, K^+, Ca^{++} and Mg^{++}; the major anions are Cl^-, HCO_3^-, HPO_4^- and protein$^-$. There are major differences between the concentration of ions in the intracellular and extracellular compartments as shown in Fig. 1.2 and Table 1.1. The major difference is in the distribution of Na^+ and K^+ with Na^+ dominating the extracellular fluid as the major cation and K^+ being the major intracellular cation.

The composition of intracellular fluid is difficult to measure and the values given in Table 1.1 are mean values calculated from the total amount of electrolyte per cell. The intracellular electrolytes are not distributed evenly throughout the cell and for example Ca^{++} is actively transported into the sarcoplasmic reticulum in skeletal muscle and the concentration of Ca^{++} in the cell water is only 0.0000001 meq/litre. There is therefore a large concentration gradient for Ca^{++} to enter the cell which is not apparent from the mean values for intracellular and extracellular Ca^{++} concentration quoted in the table.

The concentration of any electrolyte in body fluids is normally expressed in milliequivalents per litre (meq/litre). One equivalent of any electrolyte carries the same number of electrical charges as 1 gram of hydrogen ion or is 'equivalent' to 1 gram of hydrogen ion. One gram atomic weight or gram molecular weight of any substance has the same number of atoms or molecules as 1 gram of hydrogen. Therefore,

Table 1.1   Ionic composition of body water compartments

Ion	Interstitial fluid meq/litre	Intracellular fluid meq/litre
Na^+	145.1	12.0
K^+	4.4	150.0
Ca^{++}	2.4	4.0
Mg^{++}	1.1	34.0
	153.0	200.0
Cl^-	117.4	4.0
HCO_3^-	27.1	12.0
Inorganic phosphate$^-$	2.3	40.0
Organic phosphate$^-$ and other	6.2	90.0
Protein$^-$	0.0	54.0
	153.0	200.0

Source: B. D. Rose, *Clinical Physiology of Acid-Base and Electrolyte Disorders,* 2nd ed, McGraw-Hill, New York, 1984.

$$\frac{\text{atomic weight or molecular weight (in grams)}}{\text{valence}} = 1 \text{ equivalent}$$

and
$$23 \text{ mg } Na^+ = 1 \text{ mmol} = 1 \text{ meq}$$
$$40 \text{ mg } Ca^{++} = 1 \text{ mmol} = 2 \text{ meq}$$

In any solution the concentration of cations expressed in meq/litre equals the concentration of anions in meq/litre. Therefore the total concentrations of cations and anions shown in Table 1.1 balance for both extracellular and intracellular fluid. The concentrations of Na^+ and Cl^- in plasma differ slightly from those in interstitial fluid because of the presence of plasma proteins which act as a non diffusible anion in the plasma fluid compartment.

The details concerning the functions of the various electrolytes and the control mechanisms regulating their concentrations in body fluids will be given in subsequent chapters but it is useful to summarise some of the information for each ion species at this point.

Sodium

Na^+ is the major cation of the extracellular fluid and the total amount of exchangeable Na^+ determines the volume of the extracellular fluid compartment. The concentration of Na^+ determines the extracellular fluid osmolarity. Na^+ is actively transported out of cells so that the intracellular concentration of Na^+ is very low. The resting cell membrane is relatively impermeable to Na^+ but the large concentration gradient for Na^+ to move intracellularly is utilised for the generation of the action potential in nerve and muscle.

Potassium

K^+ is the major cation of the intracellular fluid. K^+ is actively transported across the cell membrane and the intracellular concentration of K^+ is much higher than that in extracellular fluid. The cell membrane of nerve and muscle is relatively permeable to K^+ and diffusion of K^+ out of the cell is responsible for the resting cell membrance potential of nerve and muscle.

Calcium

Ca^{++} is found primarily in the skeleton and teeth but its major role is as a regulator of cell metabolism and as a controller of the excitability of nerve and muscle. Ca^{++} is actively transported out of cells and there is a high concentration gradient for Ca^{++} to move from the extracellular to the intracellular compartment.

Magnesium

Mg^{++} has similar properties to Ca^{++} and is mainly found in bone and the intracellular compartment. Mg^{++} influences neuromuscular excitability and acts as an intracellular regulator of high energy phosphate production and metabolic activity.

Hydrogen

H^+ ions are formed on hydration of carbon dioxide to carbonic acid and as a by-product of metabolism of amino acids. The free H^+ concentration is several orders of magnitude less than other electrolytes such as Na^+ and is normally expressed on a log pH scale. The concentration of free H^+ determines intracellular and extracellular pH and therefore the activity of many enzyme systems.

Phosphate

Phosphate is mainly found in the skeleton and teeth as calcium phosphate and as intracellular phosphate in the form of high energy phosphates such as adenosine tri phosphate (ATP). Phosphate is also found in phospholipids and phosphoproteins which are important in maintaining the structure and function of cell membranes.

Chloride

Cl⁻ is distributed throughout the extracellular compartments as the anion accompanying Na^+ and disturbances in Na^+ balance are usually accompanied by similar changes in Cl⁻.

Bicarbonate

HCO_3^- is the anion of carbonic acid and is found primarily in the extracellular fluid compartment accompanying Na^+. The control of plasma HCO_3^- concentration via the renal system is an important regulator of blood pH.

Cell membrane potential and electrical activity

All cells have an electrical charge across their cell membrane with the inside of the cell around 1/10 of a volt negative (-90 mV) with respect to the extracellular fluid. This membrane potential is caused by diffusion of K^+ ions out of the cell down a concentration gradient as shown in Fig. 1.3.

Na^+ and K^+ are actively transported across the cell membrane and this creates a concentration gradient across the membrane for the two cations. The cell membrane is relatively permeable to K^+ and impermeable to Na^+ and therefore there is a tendency for K^+ to diffuse out of the cell and into the extracellular fluid. Only a small amount of K^+ actually leaves the cell as the outward movement of K^+ causes an inequality in the distribution of electrical charge. For each K^+ that leaves the cell an imbalanced negative anion is left in the cell and this leads to a negative electrical charge inside the cell. Negative anions do not easily follow K^+ out of the cell and neu-

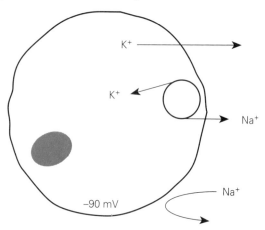

Fig. 1.3 Cell membrane potential. The cell membrane potential of –90 mV is caused by diffusion of K^+ out of the cell. The concentration gradient for K^+ is maintained by active transport of K^+ in exchange for Na^+. The resting cell membrane is relatively impermeable to Na^+.

tralise the development of a negative membrane potential as the cell membrane is impermeable to the large anions such as protein and the inward concentration gradient for Cl^- prevents much movement of Cl^- out of the cell.

The resting membrane potential of the cell is therefore determined by the concentration gradient for K^+ out of the cell and changes in the extracellular fluid concentration of K^+ have marked effects on the membrane potential.

There is a large concentration gradient as well as an electrical gradient for Na^+ to enter the cell and increases in cell permeability to Na^+ are responsible for the action potentials of nerve and muscle.

Osmolarity

The osmolarity of a solution is determined by the concentration of particles, that is the number of particles per unit volume of solvent. A particle could be an atom such as Na^+ a molecule such as glucose or a protein such as albumin, all count as one particle as far as osmolarity is concerned. The osmolarity is not influenced by the valency or size of the particles. Osmolarity is measured in osmoles/litre where the osmole is a measure of the number of particles and is therefore directly related to other units such as the mole and equivalent.

osmole = mole x n
n = number of particles molecule dissociates into

glucose (mol. wt.) 180 180 mg = 1 mmol = 1 meq = 1 mosmol
NaCl (mol. wt.) 58.5 58.5 mg = 1 mmol = 1 meq = 1.75 mosmol

Glucose is a large particle with a molecular weight of 180 and because it does not dissociate 1 mosmol is equal to 1 meq or 1 mmol. Sodium chloride dissociates into two particles Na^+ and Cl^- but the dissociation is not complete and therefore 1 meq NaCl equals 1.75 mosmol.

There is sometimes confusion between the terms 'osmolarity' and 'osmolality'

osmolarity = osmoles / litre H_2O
osmolality = osmoles / kg H_2O

In practice the difference between osmolarity and osmolality is negligible because of the very low concentrations of electrolytes in biological fluids.

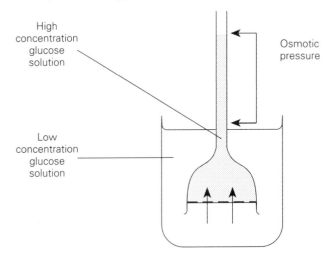

Fig. 1.4   Osmotic pressure. When a high concentration glucose solution is separated from a lower concentration glucose solution by a membrane only permeable to water the water moves through the membrane from the lower to the higher concentration glucose solution. This movement of water creates an osmotic pressure.

Osmotic pressure

If two solutions of different concentration are separated by a membrane which is permeable to water but not to solute, i.e. a semi-permeable membrane, then water moves through the membrane to the higher concentration solution. The movement of water equalises osmolarity on either side of the membrane. This movement of water can generate an osmotic pressure as illustrated in Fig. 1.4.

When discussing osmotic pressure it is important to distinguish between effective osmoles and ineffective osmoles. For example, consider the capillary wall as a semi-permeable membrane separating electrolytes in interstitial fluid and plasma. The osmolarity of plasma is 280 mosmol/litre mainly due to NaCl. If plasma was separated from water by a membrane impermeable to NaCl then it would be capable of generating an osmotic pressure of 5404 mmHg. However the capillary membrane is freely permeable to NaCl but not to plasma proteins. Therefore the net effective osmotic pressure generated across the capillary membrane is 25 mm Hg, and only relates to the plasma proteins whose concentration is 1.3 mosmol/litre. Plasma proteins are effective osmoles as they do not diffuse across the capillary whereas Na^+ and Cl^- are ineffective osmoles as they readily diffuse across the capillary.

Isotonic solutions such as 0.9% NaCl and 5% dextrose contain solute which does not readily cross cell membranes and the solutions are isosmotic with body fluids. When red blood cells are placed in an isotonic

0.9% NaCl   5% Dextrose   Isosmotic
                                          urea

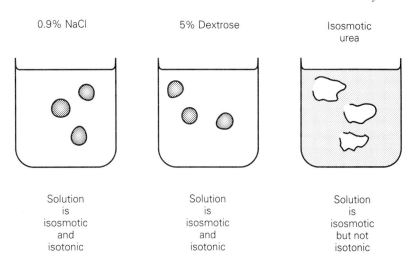

Solution   Solution   Solution
is   is   is
isosmotic   isosmotic   isosmotic
and   and   but not
isotonic   isotonic   isotonic

Fig. 1.5   Red blood cells in isosmotic solutions. Urea is an ineffective osmole for cells as it readily crosses cell membranes. Urea enters the cell and therefore the combined osmolarity of the cell is equivalent to the cell contents plus urea. The osmolarity of the cell is then greater than that of the surrounding solution of urea.Water enters the cell down an osmotic gradient and causes the cell to swell and haemolyse.

fluid there is no tendency for water to move in or out of the cell and haemolysis does not occur. However, not all isosmotic solutions are isotonic. Red blood cells placed in isosmotic urea solution haemolyse as shown in Fig. 1.5. Urea is an ineffective osmole as it readily crosses cell membranes whereas NaCl and dextrose are effective osmoles as they do not readily enter the red cell. Therefore in the red cell suspended in isosmotic urea solution urea enters the cell and the concentration of urea in the cell is similar to that of the surrounding solution. The cell osmolarity is then greater than that of the urea solution as it is equal to the cell osmoles plus urea. Water enters the cell from the urea solution and causes the cell to swell and haemolyse.

Plasma osmolarity

Water can freely pass across cell membranes and between the extracellular and intracellular compartments of the body. Therefore the osmolarity of the extracellular fluid compartment equals the osmolarity of the intracellular fluid compartment. Plasma osmolarity therefore provides a measure of the osmolarity of both extracellular and intracellular fluid compartments.

Na$^+$ and its anions Cl$^-$ and HCO$_3^-$ form the bulk of the osmoles in plasma, therefore one can estimate body osmolarity from [Na$^+$] by the formula plasma osmolarity = 2 x [Na$^+$]

                      = 2 x [142 mol/litre]

osmolarity   = 284 mosmol/litre

Body fluid osmolarity is normally around 280–290 mosmol/litre. Twice the plasma [Na$^+$] gives us a useful measure of body osmolarity. The concentrations of glucose, proteins and urea can be disregarded as contributing only a small amount to total plasma osmolarity in health.

glucose = 5 mosmol/litre

proteins = 0.9 mosmol/litre

urea   = ineffective osmole

Twice plasma [Na$^+$] gives a useful measure of plasma osmolarity as several factors tend to cancel each other out. For example, NaCl is incompletely dissociated but this is compensated by the fact that the concentration of Na$^+$ in plasma water is greater than that in whole plasma because of the dilution effect of plasma proteins. In diseases where there may be significant elevation of blood glucose or urea then the following formula is often quoted as being more clinically relevant.

plasma osmolarity = 2 x [Na$^+$ + K$^+$] + glucose + urea

The use of this formula is debatable as any rise in plasma K$^+$ is likely to prove fatal before having a significant effect on plasma osmolarity, urea is still an ineffective osmole even if its plasma concentration is elevated, and the rise in plasma osmolarity associated with hyperglycemia is mainly related to the water loss caused by an osmotic diuresis rather than a rise in blood glucose. Direct measurement of plasma osmolarity in hyperglycemic diabetes is useful as a measure of water deficit.

2　Renal function

The kidney plays a central role in the regulation of the cellular environment and renal disease causes widespread disturbances by disrupting the environment of every living cell in the body. The kidney not only filters waste products but also regulates body water and the electrolyte composition of the extracellular fluid. The kidney acts as an endocrine organ and is involved in the control of red blood cell mass via erythropoietin and the control of plasma $[Ca^{++}]$ via vitamin D metabolism. The functions of the kidney are summarised in Fig. 2.1. The main functions of the kidney concerning the regulation of electrolyte concentration and body water will be discussed in detail in later sections and only a review of functions is given in this chapter.

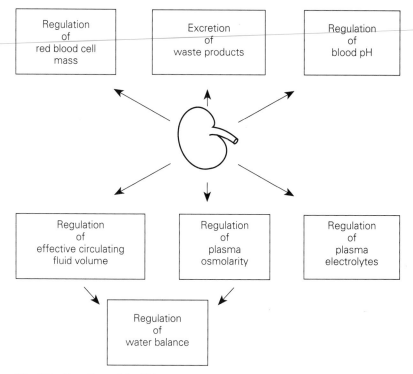

Fig. 2.1　Functions of the kidney.

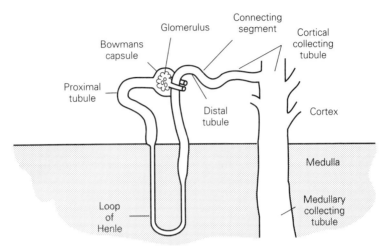

Fig.2. 2   Components of a nephron.

The functional unit of the kidney is the nephron as illustrated in Fig. 2.2 and each kidney contains over one million nephrons. A brief review of the functions of the components of the nephron is given below.

Glomerulus and Bowmans capsule

The tuft of capillaries that form the glomerulus create an ultrafiltrate from plasma which contains small molecules such as glucose, amino acids, urea and electrolytes. These substances in the ultrafiltrate are found in almost the same concentration as in the plasma. The ultrafiltrate that enters the Bowmans capsule is almost protein free as the plasma proteins are too large to pass through the glomerular filter. Filtration from the glomerular capillaries into the Bowmans capsule is determined by the hydrostatic pressure in the capillaries, around 45 mmHg, which is much higher than in systemic capillaries. The hydrostatic pressure forcing the ultrafiltrate out is opposed by the plasma osmotic pressure due to the presence of plasma proteins in the capillary but not in the capsular fluid.

The glomerular filtration rate (GFR) is around 125 ml/min and autoregulation by constriction and dilation of the afferent arteriole ensures that GFR is maintained relatively constant over a wide range of systemic arterial blood pressure (90–190 mmHg).

The kidneys receive a disproportionate percentage of the cardiac output relative to their size and renal blood flow is around 1 litre/min which is about 20% of cardiac output.

Proximal tubule

The fluid entering the proximal tubule is of a similar composition to plas-

Table 2.1 Handling of filtrate by nephron

	Proximal tubule	Loop of Henle	Distal tubule; collecting tubules
H_2O	70	5	24
NaCl	70	20	9
KCl	80	20	(secretion)
Ca^{++}	70	20	5
Mg^{++}	30	65	
HCO_3^-	90		10
Phosphates	90		
Urea	concentrated reabsorbed	recycled	concentrated reabsorbed
Glucose	100		
Amino acids	100		
Inulin	0	0	0
PAH	(secretion)		
H^+	(secretion) pH 7.4–7.0		(secretion) pH 7.0–4.5

Note: The figures, except where stated, refer to the percentage of the filtrate reabsorbed in each of the three regions of the nephron.

ma except for the absence of plasma proteins. With a GFR of 125 ml/min approximately 180 litres of plasma water are filtered into the proximal tubule each day. This means that the total plasma water passes through the kidney 60 times each day. Of the 180 litres of plasma water filtered each day only around 1.5 litres is lost as urine and the remaining 178.5 litres of fluid is reabsorbed by the nephron.

The proximal tubule plays a very important role in the reabsorption of filtrate as approximately 70% of the solute and water in the filtrate is absorbed by the proximal tubule. The proximal tubule is particularly involved in reabsorbing the majority of the filtered water, Na^+, K^+, Cl^-, HCO_3^-, phosphate, glucose and amino acids as shown in Table 2.1.

Special points to note about the figures quoted for the proximal tubule in Table 2.1 are that:

1. The major osmole in the ultrafiltrate is Na^+ and since 70% of Na^+ is reabsorbed by the proximal tubule 70% of the water follows this solute down an osmotic gradient.
2. Urea is concentrated in the proximal tubule when the filtered solute and water are reabsorbed and urea is left behind. Because of the high solubility of urea, it readily crosses the renal tubule and is passively reabsorbed when the concentration of urea in the tubule exceeds that in the renal capillaries.
3. All of the glucose and amino acids in the filtrate are reabsorbed by the proximal tubule.

4. Substances such as para-amino hippuric acid (PAH) are actively secreted into the proximal renal tubule.
5. Although the pH of the fluid in the proximal tubule only changes from pH 7.4 to 7.0 this involves a large amount of H^+ secretion. Ninety per cent of the filtered HCO_3^- is reabsorbed in the proximal tubule and this involves reaction of HCO_3^- with secreted H^+. Probably more than 90% of the total H^+ secreted by the nephron is secreted in the proximal tubule but the pH change is buffered on filtered HCO_3^-.

The mechanisms involved in reabsorption of water and solute in the proximal tubule are diagrammed in Fig. 2.3. Na^+ is the major osmole in the filtrate and Na^+ readily enters the renal tubular cell down an electrochemical gradient. The concentration of Na^+ is low in the tubular cell and the membrane potential is around -70 mv. Both these factors favour movement of Na^+ inside the cell. Na^+ is actively pumped from the tubular cell on the capillary side in exchange for K^+. Na^+ is also actively transported into the intercellular spaces, Cl^- follows to maintain electroneutrality, and H_2O follows the osmotic gradient. Na^+ is also transported in exchange for H^+. The H^+ secretion is important for reabsorption of HCO_3^- from the tubular fluid and 90% of filtered HCO_3^- is reabsorbed in the proximal tubule.

Most of the filtered K^+ is reabsorbed by the proximal tubule but the mechanism is not known as K^+ must move into the cell against a high concentration gradient. K^+ may be reabsorbed in exchange for H^+ secretion.

All of the filtered amino acids, glucose and nearly all phosphates are reabsorbed by the proximal tubule. The concentration gradient for Na^+ to enter the tubular cell is utilised for passive co-transport of amino acids, glucose and phosphates and these leave the cell by facilitated diffusion.

As solute and water are reabsorbed so urea is concentrated in the tubule. Urea readily penetrates cell membranes and some is reabsorbed by the proximal tubule. Urea excretion depends on a good flow of urine as urea is passively washed out with the urine flow.

Ca^{++} is passively reabsorbed across the luminal membrane of the tubule as the filtrate is concentrated by reabsorption of NaCl and H_2O. Active transport of Ca^{++} may occur across the peritubular membrane in exchange for Na^+.

The proximal tubule has secretory mechanisms for organic acids and bases such as para-amino hippuric acid (PAH), penicillin and histamine and these substances are actively secreted from the renal capillaries into the filtrate.

Loop of Henle

The function of the loop of Henle is to create a hyperosmotic environment in the renal medulla. The osmolarity of the renal medulla may reach 900–1400 mosmol/litre as compared to a plasma osmolarity of 280–290

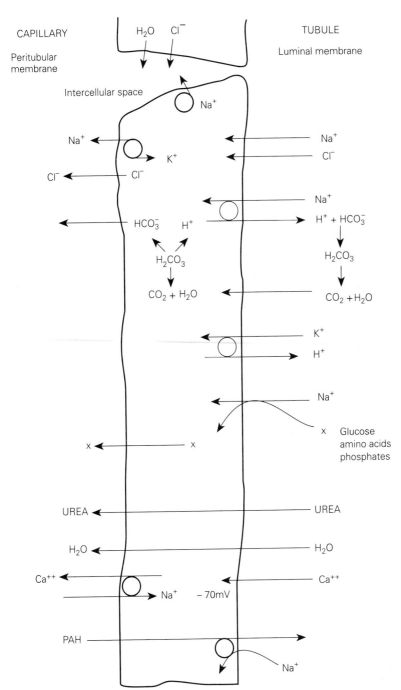

Fig. 2.3 Proximal tubule, mechanisms for reabsorption of water and solute.

mosmol/litre. The osmotic gradient created by the loop of Henle is utilised by the collecting tubules for concentration of urine. The maximum osmolarity of the urine is therefore determined by the osmotic gradient created by the loop of Henle.

The loop of Henle creates the osmotic gradient in the medulla by active transport of NaCl from the ascending limb as illustrated in Fig. 2.4. Cl^- is actively transported out of the tubule and Na^+ follows passively. The two limbs of the loop differ in their permeability to water as the descending limb is relatively permeable to water and the ascending limb relatively impermeable. Active transport of NaCl from the ascending limb creates an osmotic gradient for water to leave the descending limb. As fluid moves down the descending limb the osmolarity increases up to 1400

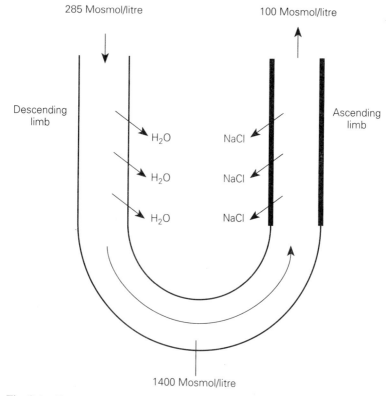

Fig. 2.4   Counter-current multiplier of loop of Henle. The descending limb of the loop of Henle is relatively impermeable to solute but permeable to water therefore water leaves the tubule into the medulla. The ascending limb actively transports NaCl into the medulla and is relatively impermeable to water. Active transport of NaCl creates the osmotic gradient for water to leave the descending limb. As fluid descends the loop loss of water increases the osmolarity and as fluid enters the ascending limb loss of NaCl decreases osmolarity.

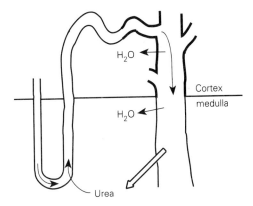

Fig. 2.5 Recycling of urea. Water reabsorption from the collecting tubule concentrates urea in the tubular fluid. The inner medullary collecting tubule is relatively permeable to urea and the concentrated urea escapes into the medulla. Urea can then enter the loop of Henle and be recycled to maintain the medullary osmotic gradient.

mosmol/litre and as it moves up the ascending limb osmolarity decreases due to loss of NaCl.

This mechanism of creating the osmotic gradient is termed a countercurrent multiplier as the loop creates flows in opposite directions and the limbs of the loop are close enough to influence each other.

Only half of the 1400 mosmol/litre osmotic gradient in the renal medulla is related to NaCl and the other half is related to urea which is trapped and recycled around the medulla as illustrated in Fig. 2.5. In the presence of anti-diuretic hormone (ADH) the collecting tubules of the cortex and medulla are permeable to water. Water leaves the collecting tubules down an osmotic gradient and urea is concentrated in the cortical collecting tubule due to its relative impermeability for urea. The inner medullary collecting tubule is permeable to urea and the concentrated urea escapes into the medullary interstitial space. Urea may readily penetrate the loop of Henle and be recycled. The recycling of urea contributes half the osmolarity of the medulla but because of the small volume of the medullary interstitial space, only a tiny amount of the filtered load of urea is trapped in this space.

Unlike other capillaries in the body the medullary capillaries (vasa recta) are hairpin or looped like the loop of Henle. The capillaries are freely permeable to water and solute but because of exchange between the ascending and descending limbs of the capillary the osmotic gradient in the medulla is not disrupted. If the capillaries ran straight through the medulla the medullary osmotic gradient would be washed away. This mechanism which maintains the osmotic gradient is termed counter current exchange as the looped capillary creates flows in opposite directions with exchange of water and solute between the limbs.

The figures for filtrate reabsorption in Table 2.1 show that 20% of filtered NaCl is reabsorbed from the loop of Henle but only 5% of the filtered water. The fluid entering the loop of Henle from the proximal tubule is isosmotic with plasma (285 mosmol/litre) but fluid leaving the ascending limb of the loop is markedly hyposmotic (100 mosmol/litre). The final osmolarity of the urine is determined by water and NaCl reabsorption from the cortical and medullary collecting tubules and not by the loop of Henle.

The majority of filtered Mg^{++} is reabsorbed by the loop of Henle, unlike other electrolytes where the majority of reabsorption occurs in the proximal tubule. The regulation of Mg^{++} reabsorption is poorly understood and may involve a direct effect of Mg^{++} on the renal tubule.

Distal tubule, connecting segment, collecting tubules

The distal tubule and connecting segment absorb around 5% of the filtered NaCl, but are relatively impermeable to water. Therefore the osmolarity of the fluid leaving the loop of Henle is lowered from 100 mosm/litre to around 50–75 mosmol/litre. This represents the minimum osmolarity of urine. The distal tubule and connecting segment are not influenced by the hormones aldosterone and ADH and the amount of NaCl reabsorbed is directly proportional to the amount delivered to the segment.

The collecting tubules determine the final composition of the urine as regards Na^+, K^+, H_2O and H^+ content. The great majority of solute and water is reabsorbed in the proximal tubule, loop of Henle and distal tubule prior to reaching the collecting tubule. The collecting tubule rather than dealing with the bulk of the glomerular filtrate exerts fine control over solute and water balance in the body.

The mechanisms involved in the reabsorption/secretion of solute and water in the collecting tubule are shown in Fig. 2.6. The collecting tubule regulates Na^+ and K^+ balance under the influence of the hormone aldosterone. Aldosterone causes an increase in Na^+ reabsorption in the collecting tubule by increasing the permeability of the luminal membrane to Na^+ and by stimulating the activity of the peritubular Na^+/K^+ pump. Aldosterone increases K^+ secretion by causing an increased permeability of the luminal membrane to K^+ which facilitates movement of K^+ down a concentration gradient from the cell into the tubule. The great majority (85%) of NaCl is reabsorbed by Na^+ entering the cell down a concentration gradient and Cl^- following to maintain electrical neutrality.

Na^+ is also reabsorbed in exchange for H^+ and this mechanism is stimulated by aldosterone. As will be explained later in the section on acid base balance, if Cl^- is not available for reabsorption with Na^+ then more H^+ secretion occurs in exchange for Na^+.

K^+ secretion is passive and depends on movement of K^+ out of the cell

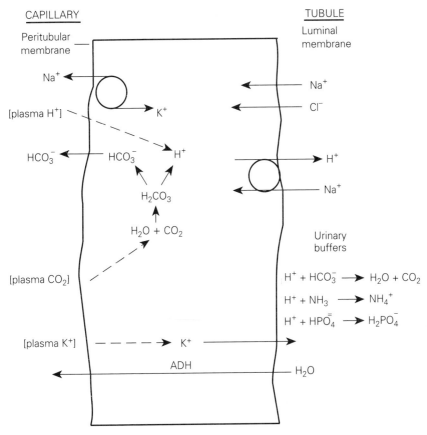

Fig. 2.6 Collecting tubule mechanisms for reabsorption/secretion of solute and water.

down a concentration gradient. K^+ secretion is increased when there is a rise in plasma $[K^+]$ as this increases the entry of K^+ into the renal tubular cell. A high plasma $[K^+]$ will also stimulate release of aldosterone from the adrenal cortex and aldosterone causes an increased permeability of the luminal membrane to K^+. Because the movement of K^+ out of the renal tubular cell is passive an increased flow of urine due to diuretic treatment will tend to wash out K^+ from the tubular cells. Therefore the use of diuretics can lead to hypokalaemia.

The final pH and $[H^+]$ of the urine is determined by H^+ secretion from the collecting tubule. When plasma $[H^+]$ and PCO_2 are elevated these influence the intracellular $[H^+]$ as illustrated in Fig. 2.6. Acidaemia and hypercapnia stimulate H^+ secretion from the collecting tubule and cause the formation of an acid urine. H^+ secretion generates HCO_3^- by hydration of CO_2 as shown in Fig. 2.6. The rate of formation of carbonic acid in the renal tubular cell is increased by the presence of carbonic anhydrase. The majority of the H^+ secreted by the collecting tubule are buffered on HCO_3^-, NH_3 and $HPO_4^=$ and the presence of these urinary buffers greatly increase the capacity for H^+ secretion.

The osmolarity of the urine and body water balance are controlled by the collecting tubule under the influence of ADH. In the absence of ADH the collecting tubule is relatively impermeable to water and the hypo-osmotic fluid delivered from the distal tubule is excreted with an osmolarity of 75–100 mosmol/litre. Absence of ADH causes diuresis with the formation of a large volume of hypo-osmotic urine. In the presence of ADH the collecting tubule is permeable to water and water is reabsorbed along an osmotic gradient into the cortex and medulla as illustrated in Fig. 2.7. Fluid leaving the ascending limb of the loop of Henle is hypoosmotic to plasma (100 mosmol/litre) and in the presence of ADH water leaves the cortical collecting tubule down an osmotic gradient. Reabsorption of water in the cortical collecting tubule is important as it allows the medullary collecting tubules to concentrate a smaller volume of urine. As the fluid passes down the medullary collecting tubule it is exposed to the osmotic gradient created by the loop of Henle. The fluid can then be concentrated by reabsorption of water along an osmotic gradient up to a final urine osmolarity of 1400 mosmol/litre.

Hormonal control of renal function

The role of hormones in the control of Na^+ and H_2O balance will be discussed in more detail in later sections but it is useful to summarise some information at this point. A summary of hormonal control is given in Fig. 2.8. ADH secreted from the posterior pituitary controls water balance by increasing the permeability of the collecting tubules to water and thus promoting water retention. Aldosterone secreted from the adrenal cortex stimulates Na^+ reabsorption and K^+ secretion at the level of the collecting tubules. Atrial natriuretic peptide (ANP) is another hormone involved in Na^+ balance and is stored in the walls of the atria and released in response to atrial stretch. The natriuretic effect of ANP is mainly caused by an increase in glomerular filtration rate (GFR) causing an increased filtered load of Na^+ and Na^+ loss in urine. Parathyroid hormone (PTH) released from the parathyroid gland causes an increased Ca^{++} reabsorption at the level of the distal tubule and connecting segment. PTH also increases phosphate loss in urine by decreasing phosphate reabsorption at the proximal tubule. H^+ secretion and HCO_3^- reabsorption are not under hormonal control and are directly influenced by plasma $[H^+]$ and plasma P CO_2. The excretion of urea is mainly determined by the rate of urine flow as urea is passively reabsorbed and concentrated along the renal tubule.

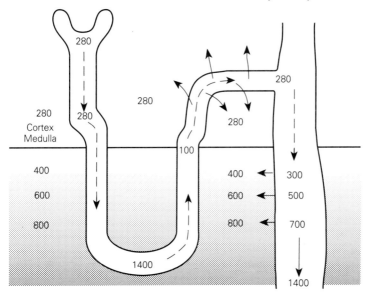

Fig. 2.7 Effect of ADH on collecting tubule. The nephron is illustrated in diagramatic form and the numbers relate to osmolarity in mosmol/litre. The arrows indicate movement of water from the cortical and medullary collecting tubules under the influence of ADH.

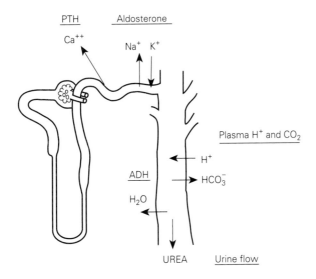

Fig. 2.8 Hormonal control of renal function.

Glomerular filtration rate

Glomerular filtration rate (GFR) is an important parameter of renal function, especially in determining the severity of renal failure in clinical practice. The GFR is the rate at which the kidneys filter plasma and normal
GFR is around 125 ml/min. GFR can be used as a measure of functioning
renal mass and for example the loss of one kidney will cause an acute 50%
reduction in GFR.

GFR can be estimated by measuring the rate at which some marker substance is filtered by the kidneys. If one knows the amount of substance
filtered each minute and the plasma concentration of the substance then
GFR or the rate at which plasma is filtered can be calculated. This estimate
of GFR is termed clearance as it measures the rate at which plasma is
cleared of the substance.

$$\text{clearance ml/min} = \frac{\text{amount of substance filtered / min}}{\text{plasma concentration / ml}}$$

The amount of substance filtered each minute can be determined by
urine collection assuming that the substance is filtered but not secreted,
reabsorbed or synthesised by the kidney. An assumption is also made that
the plasma concentration is steady state. The conventional formula for
clearance of a substance is

$$Cx = \frac{Ux \times V}{Px}$$

where
    Cx = clearance of substance x in ml/min
    Ux = amount of x in urine
    V = urine flow in ml/min
    Px = plasma concentration per ml

Clearance is independent of the plasma concentration of the substance.
The higher the concentration in plasma the more substance is filtered each
minute, however the volume of plasma cleared of the substance each
minute remains constant as shown in Fig. 2.9.

The graph shown in Fig. 2.9 would be applicable to inulin, a polysac-
charide which is filtered by the kidney but which is not reabsorbed, secreted or synthesised by the kidney. Inulin is the classical substance used to
determine clearance experimentally but it is not used clinically to assess
renal function as an intravenous infusion of inulin is required and this
method would be too time-consuming for routine clinical assesment of
renal function.

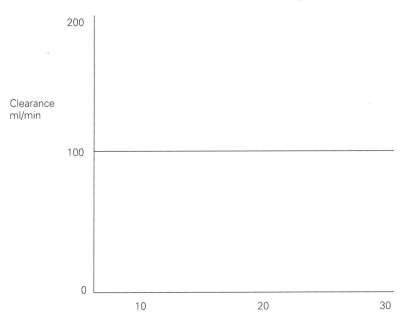

Fig. 2.9 Clearance and plasma concentration. Clearance of a substance such as inulin,which is neither reabsorbed, secreted or synthesised by the kidney is independent of the plasma concentration of the substance.

Creatinine clearance (Ccr) or more commonly the plasma concentration of creatinine (Pcr) is used clinically as a measure of renal function. Creatinine is a waste product of muscle metabolism and is released at a steady rate from metabolising skeletal muscle. The plasma concentration of creatinine is determined primarily by muscle mass if renal function is normal. Renal disease which affects GFR causes an increase in plasma creatinine concentration. The plasma concentration of creatinine reaches a steady state level depending on the balance between creatinine production by skeletal muscle and renal clearance of creatinine as shown in Fig. 2.10.

Since there is an equilibrium between creatinine production and renal clearance of creatinine the plasma creatinine concentration varies inversely with GFR. If GFR goes down with renal failure then creatinine accumulates in the blood and measurement of plasma creatinine concentration itself will give an estimate of renal function and GFR. Plasma creatinine concentration should be measured in a fasting subject as a meat meal will elevate the plasma level of creatinine by as much as 50%.

Plasma creatinine concentration is influenced by the effects of age, weight and sex on body muscle mass, and in clinical use the measurement

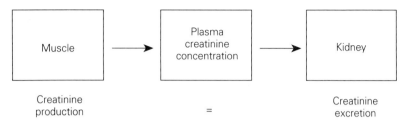

Fig. 2.10 The plasma creatinine concentration is determined by a balance between creatinine production from skeletal muscle and creatinine loss via the kidneys. Plasma creatinine concentration can be a useful measure of renal function as a decrease in GFR will lead to elevation of plasma creatinine concentration.

of plasma creatinine can only provide a rough guide to the adequacy of renal function. Creatinine clearance can be calculated from the clearance formula using plasma creatinine concentration and a 24-hour urine sample and this gives a much more reliable measure of renal function. The major error involved in determining creatinine clearance is incomplete urine collection and this should be suspected if the the total amount of creatinine excreted in 24 hours is much less than the normal predicted value.

Urea is excreted by the kidneys and it accumulates in the blood on renal failure. Urea clearance is not a useful measure of renal function as there are many factors that influence urea production and excretion independent of GFR. Unlike creatinine the production of urea is not constant and is mainly determined by the rate of hepatic metabolism of amino acids. A high protein diet, trauma or bleeding into the digestive tract can all increase the production of urea. Only half the filtered urea is excreted in the urine and urea reabsorption tends to passively follow NaCl reabsorption. The plasma concentration of urea is increased with dehydration as the urea is concentrated in the remaining volume of body water and the renal water retention caused by ADH also causes retention of urea. Creatinine clearance is not affected to the same extent by dehydration as the creatinine filtered by the kidney is not reabsorbed. A persistently elevated plasma creatinine concentration is therefore the first indicator of renal disease and this can be confirmed by measuring creatinine clearance.

3 Regulation of effective circulating volume

Adequate tissue perfusion is essential for the maintenance of a cellular environment compatible with life. The perfusion of the tissues is primarily determined by cardiac output and systemic vascular resistance but in order for the blood to be moved through the capillaries there must also be an adequate blood volume. If blood volume is decreased due to a decrease in extracellular fluid caused by dehydration or blood loss then tissue perfusion will be affected due to a decrease in cardiac output.

The perfusion of the tissues is related to both both cardiac output and extracellular fluid volume but this relationship is complex. Cardiac output and extracellular fluid volume can be measured but the vital parameter which is the volume of fluid that is effectively perfusing the tissues cannot be measured. The *effective circulating volume* refers to that part of the extracellular fluid contained in the vascular space which is effectively perfusing the tissues. Effective perfusion involves blood flow through the capillaries as this allows exchange of gases, nutrients and metabolites between the tissues and the blood.

Effective circulating volume is a concept, an idea. It is related to blood volume and extracellular fluid volume but both of these volumes may vary independently of effective circulating volume. For example, in hypovolaemia blood volume is reduced and so is effective circulating volume but in cardiac failure blood volume is normal or increased and effective circulating volume is reduced. Congestive heart failure results in a decrease in effective circulating volume with an increase in extracellular fluid volume. Vasovagal syncope is associated with a decrease in effective circulating volume yet extracellular fluid volume is unchanged.

The consequences of a decrease in effective circulating volume and the cardiovascular and renal compensatory responses are discussed in the section on cardiovascular shock. There is some overlap between these sections but the present section deals with the physiological mechanisms rather than the clinical condition of cardiovascular shock.

How are changes in effective circulating volume sensed

Adequate perfusion of the peripheral circulation is vital but there are no sensors which directly sense the effective circulating volume. If there were blood flow detectors throughout the peripheral circulation the effective circulating volume could be monitored by the rate of perfusion of the peripheral circulation. Blood flow detectors do not exist in the circulation and instead the stretching or pressure in sensitive regions of the cardiovascular system provides information about effective circulating volume. Pressure and volume are directly related and therefore pressure changes detected at various renal and extra renal sites provide information about effective circulating volume. The locations of these sites acting as sensors for pressure and volume are illustrated in Fig. 3.1.

Changes in arterial blood pressure are detected by the barroceptors of the carotid sinus and aortic arch. Blood pressure provides a pressure head for perfusion of the peripheral circulation and a fall in arterial blood pressure can reduce effective circulating volume. Taken to extremes when blood pressure falls to zero, effective circulating volume is also zero as no blood would flow through the peripheral circulation. We cannot measure effective circulating volume as a parameter and determine a relationship

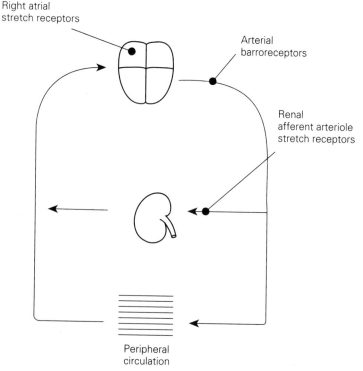

Fig. 3.1 Sensors detecting changes in effective circulating volume. Effective circulating volume cannot be sensed directly but stretch or pressure changes in the cardiovascular system provide indirect information about the perfusion of the peripheral circulation.

with blood pressure, but it is self-evident that any uncompensated fall in arterial blood pressure will decrease the rate of perfusion of the peripheral circulation.

The filling of the cardiovascular circuit is detected by stretch receptors in the right atrium. Increased stretching of the atrium is related to increased filling due to increased venous return or venous pressure. Hypovolaemia due to haemorrhage causes decreases in venous return, venous pressure and filling of the right atrium.

The perfusion of the kidney is influenced by changes in effective circulating volume. Stretch receptors in the afferent arteriole detect changes in renal perfusion caused by fluctuations in arterial pressure.

Stimulation of the sensors described above and illustrated in Fig. 3.1 cause changes in nervous and hormonal activity which in turn influence the cardiovascular and renal systems and bring about changes in effective circulating volume.

Arterial barroreceptor reflex

The arterial barroreceptors detect changes in arterial blood pressure and bring about reflex changes in cardiac output and peripheral resistance. The arterial barroreceptors are stretch or pressure receptors located in the walls of the cartoid and aortic arteries. The sensory nerves supplying the barroreceptors join the vagus and glossopharyngeal nerves to enter the brain at the level of the medulla oblongata. The barroreceptors are stimulated by a rise in arterial blood pressure. Changes in arterial blood pressure cause reflex changes in the autonomic nerves controlling the heart and total peripheral resistance particularly the sympathetic nerves to the heart and blood vessels as illustrated in Fig. 3.2.

Stimulation of arterial barroreceptors inhibits sympathetic nervous activity. A fall in arterial blood pressure therefore releases the sympathetic nervous system from this inhibitory input and causes tachycardia and vasoconstriction which tend to raise blood pressure back towards normal. These responses are discussed in more detail in the section on cardiovascular shock. In general arterial vasoconstriction raises total peripheral resistance and causes a shunting of blood flow from skin, gut and kidney towards the heart, lungs and brain. Venoconstriction increases venous return and perfusion of the peripheral circulation by squeezing blood from the large capacitance veins into the peripheral circulation. Over two thirds of the total blood volume is contained within the venous circulation and this large volume of blood can be considered as a 'spare tank' of blood which can be squeezed into the circulation when required. Sympathetic stimulation of the heart causes tachycardia accompanied by an increased force of contraction and this results in an increased cardiac output.

The sympathetic nervous response to barroreceptor activity is rapid and occurs in a few seconds. This cardiovascular response is the first line of defence in maintaining effective circulating volume and it ensures ade-

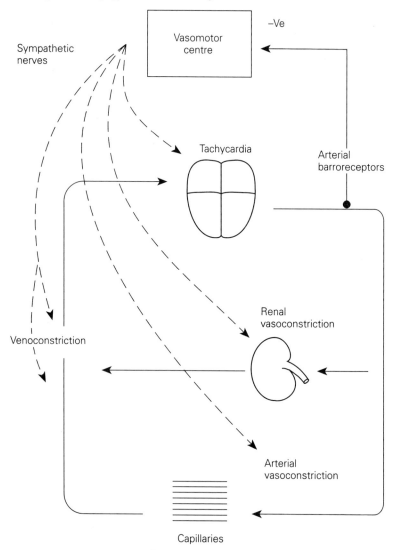

Fig. 3.2   Barroreceptor reflex. Stimulation of arterial barroreceptors inhibits sympathetic nervous activity. A fall in arterial blood pressure therefore releases sympathetic activity from this inhibitory activity and causes tachycardia and vasoconstriction.

quate perfusion of the vital organs when effective circulating volume is rapidly decreased as for example with hypovolaemia due to haemorrhage.

Changes in arterial barroreceptor activity can also influence the release of renin from the kidney and ADH from the pituitary. The increased sympathetic vasoconstrictor activity caused by a fall in arterial blood pressure stimulates renin release from the juxta glomerular apparatus of the nephron. The barroreceptor input to the brainstem areas also influences ADH release and a fall in blood pressure increases ADH release from the pituitary.

Right atrial stretch receptor reflex

Stretch receptors located in the wall of the right atrium have been shown to influence the release of ADH from the pituitary. The stretch receptors are supplied by sensory branches of the vagus nerve. Increased filling and stretching of the right atrium has been shown to cause a diuresis by inhibition of ADH and similarly decreased filling causes an increase in ADH secretion and renal water retention as illustrated in Fig. 3.3. Hypovolaemia causes a decreased filling and stretching of the right atrium which causes an increase in ADH secretion and water retention. Increased blood levels of ADH cause water retention by increasing the permeability of the renal collecting tubules to water. ADH release is primarily controlled by osmoreceptors and changes in ADH release regulate body fluid osmolarity. However, there are circumstances when there may be a conflict between osmoregulation and volume regulation and in these instances preservation of blood volume takes priority. In animal experiments only a very slight haemorrhage is sufficent to abolish a renal diuresis caused by infusion of hypotonic fluids.

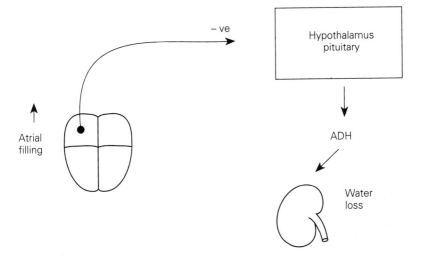

Fig. 3.3   Atrial stretch receptor reflex. Increased filling and stretch of the atria inhibits ADH release from the pituitary and causes water loss with a diuresis. Decreased filling of the atria as might occur with haemmorrhage, has the opposite action and causes an increase in ADH release and water retention.

The cardiac atria as well as acting as a pump also have an endocrine function. Atrial natriuretic hormone has been shown to be released in response to increased filling and stretch of the atria. Atrial natriuretic hormone causes increased renal loss of Na^+ by decreasing Na^+ reabsorption. The existence of an atrial natriuretic hormone helps to explain why excessive secretion of the hormone aldosterone does not cause an excessive increase in extracellular fluid volume. Primary hyperaldosteronism with increased levels of aldosterone is not usually associated with oedema and excessive increase in extracellular fluid. This 'escape' from the actions of aldosterone which stimulates Na^+ reabsorption may be due to the antagonistic effects of atrial natriuretic hormone which limits any increase in extracellular fluid and blood volume. In contrast congestive heart disease with aldosterone excess is associated with oedema and accumulation of extracellular fluid. Perhaps disruption of atrial natriuretic hormone release from the atria contributes to the development of oedema.

Renal response to changes in effective circulating volume

Extracellular fluid volume is determined by total body stores of Na^+ since Na^+ is the major extracellular osmole. Therefore regulation of Na^+ balance by the kidney plays an important role in regulating effective circulating volume. Plasma Na^+ concentration determines extracellular fluid osmolarity but plasma Na^+ concentration varies independently from total body stores of Na^+. Both hyponatrenia and hypernatraemia may be associated with normal body stores of Na^+ and in these disorders it is the ratio of Na^+ stores to body water that is changed not necessarily the absolute amounts of Na^+ or water.

Changes in effective circulating volume are detected by stretch receptors in the afferent arteriole to the nephron and possibly by the cells of the macula densa in the distal tube which detect changes in NaCl delivery. The Bowmans capsule lies next to the distal renal tubule and the afferent and efferent arterioles wrap around the distal tubule. This arrangement is termed the juxta glomerular apparatus. The afferent arteriole contains specialised smooth muscle cells called juxta glomerular cells which secrete the proteolytic enzyme renin. Renin is released in response to renal hypoperfusion (decreased arteriolar stretch) and also in response to increased sympathetic nervous activity. Renin acts on a plasma substance angiotensinogen to form angiotensin I which is converted to angiotensin II in the lungs. Angiotensin II has several actions:

1. causes aldosterone release from the adrenal cortex;
2. directly stimulates Na^+, H_2O reabsorption in renal tubule;
3. acts as a potent vasoconstrictor;
4. enhances the sensitivity of blood vessels to noradrenaline;
5. stimulates thirst.

The main control of the renin-angiotensin system is via Na$^+$ intake as high Na$^+$ intake expands extracellular volume and decreases renin release, and a low Na$^+$ intake leads to volume depletion and increases renin release. Hypovolaemia is a potent stimulus for renin release and here the increased sympathetic nervous activity to the kidney causing renal vaso-constriction may also directly stimulate renin release from the juxta glomerular cells of the afferent arteriole. The renal response to hypo-volaemia/hypotension is illustrated in Fig. 3.4.

Hypovolaemia stimulates renal Na$^+$ reabsorption as described above and

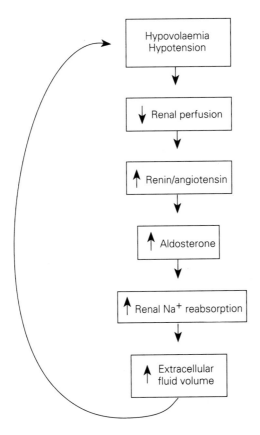

Fig. 3.4 Renal response to changes in effective circulating volume. A decrease in effective circulating volume associated with hypovolaemia/hypotension causes a decrease in renal perfusion which stimulates renin release. Renin causes formation of angiotensin I and II and stimulation of aldosterone release from the adrenal cor-tex. Aldosterone stimulates renal reabsorption of Na$^+$ which leads to an increase in extracellular fluid volume which tends to restore blood volume and blood pressure back towards normal.

illustrated in Fig. 3.4 but in order for blood volume and extracellular volume to expand the Na$^+$ retention must be accompanied by water retention. Na$^+$ retention will tend to cause hypernatraemia and an increase in plasma osmolarity but this is limited as any increase in plasma osmolarity stimulates osmoreceptors in the hypothalamus and causes ADH release.

ADH stimulates renal reabsorption of water and water retention. Thirst accompanies ADH release and the sensation of thirst may also be stimulated by increased levels of angiotensin II. Thirst increases water intake, and ADH causes water retention. The increase in body water together with Na$^+$ retention, combine to expand extracellular fluid volume.

Combined cardiovascular-renal response

A decrease in effective circulating volume due to hypovolaemia/hypotension causes a combined cardiovascular and renal response. If the hypovolaemia is primarily related to decreased Na$^+$ intake then the renal response may dominate with aldosterone regulating a renal increase in Na$^+$ reabsorption. On a day-to-day basis, secretion of aldosterone and natriuretic hormone are probably the main regulators of effective circulating volume. With hypovolaemia due to haemorrhage the cardiovascular response dominates and tachycardia and vasoconstriction maintain the effective circulating volume and ensure adequate perfusion of the vital circulations. In the long term, recovery from haemorrhage requires a renal response to restore extracellular fluid volume.

The combined cardiovascular and renal responses to hypovolaemia /hypotension are illustrated in Fig. 3.5. The cardiovascular response of vasoconstriction and tachycardia tends to maintain peripheral ciculation through the heart, lungs and brain at the expense of a reduced circulation through skin and gut. The renal response develops more slowly as time is required for the full development of the hormonal response from the kidney which retains Na$^+$ and H$_2$O to expand the extracellular fluid volume back to normal.

Summary

Effective circulating volume is a concept and not a parameter that can be measured. Effective circulating volume is related to extracellular fluid volume and the factors influencing the perfusion of the peripheral circulation, but it is not directly related to any one paramter such as blood volume or arterial blood pressure.

Changes in effective circulating volume are detected indirectly by arterial barroreceptors, atrial stretch receptors and changes in renal perfusion. These sensors trigger reflex cardiovascular and renal responses through increased sympathetic nervous activity and increased secretions of ADH

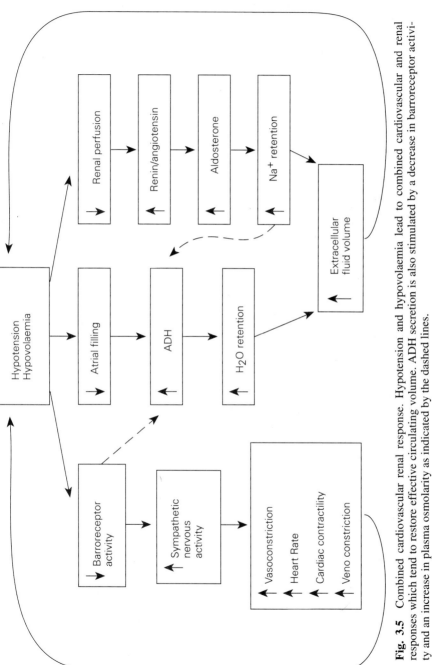

Fig. 3.5 Combined cardiovascular renal response. Hypotension and hypovolaemia lead to combined cardiovascular and renal responses which tend to restore effective circulating volume. ADH secretion is also stimulated by a decrease in barroreceptor activity and an increase in plasma osmolarity as indicated by the dashed lines.

and aldosterone. The combined cardiovascular and renal responses maintain the peripheral circulation and restore extracellular fluid volume when effective circulating volume is decreased by hypovolaemia and hypotension.

4 Regulation of plasma osmolarity and water balance

The plasma [Na^+] is the main factor determining plasma osmolarity. As discussed in Chapter 1, a good measure of plasma osmolarity is twice the plasama [Na^+] concentration since Na^+ and its salts form the bulk of the electrolytes in extracellular fluid. It is not the total amount of exchangeable Na^+ that determines plasma osmolarity but the ratio between total body water and total body Na^+. Total body Na^+ content determines extracellular fluid volume and this has been previously discussed in relation to effective circulating volume. Plasma osmolarity could theoretically be regulated by changes in Na^+ intake and excretion, if body water content was fixed. However, it is the intake and loss of water rather than changes in Na^+ balance which determines plasma osmolarity.

Normal plasma osmolarity is regulated in the range 280–290 mosmol/litre by secretion of ADH from the pituitary gland. The osmotic threshold for ADH release is around 282 mosmol/litre and with a normal plasma osmolarity of about 286 mosmol/litre plasma ADH concentration is 2–3 pg/ml and urine osmolarity 300–400 mosmol/litre. Changes in plasma osmolarity of as little as plus or minus 2% can cause maximum concentration or dilution of urine via changes in ADH secretion. Marked changes in plasma osmolarity can produce severe neurologic disorder and coma but with free access to water and normal renal function the plasma osmolarity is kept remarkably constant over a wide range of water intake. Disorders of osmolarity are much more likely to occur in the unconscious patient who cannot control water intake or in the patient with renal disease where the capacity of the kidney to concentrate urine is limited.

Plasma osmolarity is determined by a balance between water intake and water loss:

$$\frac{\text{Water intake}}{\text{regulated by thirst}} = \frac{\text{Water loss}}{\text{regulated by ADH secretion}}$$

Both the thirst mechanism and ADH secretion are regulated by osmoreceptors in the hypothalamus. Over a period of time water intake must balance water loss if plasm osmolarity is to remain within the normal range.

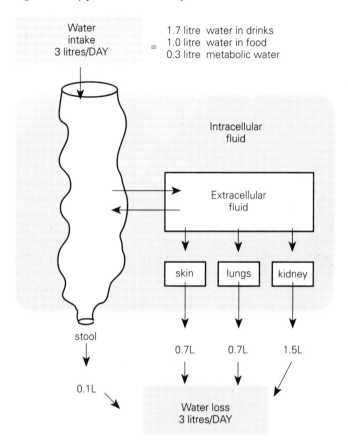

Water
intake   1.7 litre water in drinks
3 litres/DAY = 1.0 litre water in food
                0.3 litre metabolic water

Intracellular fluid

Extracellular fluid

skin   lungs   kidney

stool

0.1L

0.7L   0.7L   1.5L

Water loss
3 litres/DAY

Fig. 4.1 Daily water balance. Water intake of three litres balances water loss from gut, skin, lungs and kidney. There is a great flux of water across the digestive tract as water is absorbed and as water enters the digestive tract as secretions.

Water-balance

Water intake balances water loss over a period of time and the sources of intake and loss are illustrated in Fig. 4.1. Normal water intake is very much influenced by climate, activity, diet and social factors. Much of our water intake is related to habit rather than thirst with most intake related to meals or tea/coffee breaks.

If a normal water intake is accepted as around three litres each day then around half of this would be taken as drink and the other half as water in food and metabolic water. Most foods contain a lot of water and some fruits are close to 99% water. Normal body metabolism with oxidation of carbohydrates and fats produces around 0.3 litre water each day and this can be considered as part of water intake.

In order to maintain water balance the three litres of water intake must be matched by three litres of water loss. Around half the water is lost in the urine and half via the skin and lungs. Only a little water is normally lost in the stool but with diarrhoea this can be greatly increased. Around 0.7 litres of water is lost each day through the respiratory system by humidification of inspired air and a similar amount is lost through the skin as insensible loss. These respiratory and skin losses can be greatly increased with exercise in a hot climate and under these conditions sweat loss alone can reach up to a maximum of 1.5 litre/hr.

Water intake into the gut is shown in Fig. 4.1 as 2.7 litre/day but there is a great flux of water and solute across the gut each day related to the digestive secretions and this is illustrated in Fig. 4.2. The water contained in the digestive secretions each day comprise 20% of total body water at around six to eight litres a day. The digestive secretions contain electolytes, and over one day a significant fraction of the total body electrolytes enters the digestive tract, with 25% of total body exchangeable Na^+, 34% of exchangeable Cl^- and 3% of exchangeable K^+ entering the digestive tract each day as illustrated in Fig. 4.2. Three per cent of exchangeable K^+ does not at first appear to be a large fraction of the K^+ content. However, it does represent over 30% of the total K^+ in extracellular fluid and loss of K^+ in digestive secretions can cause severe hypokalaemia. Obviously, diarrhoea or drainage of digestive secretions

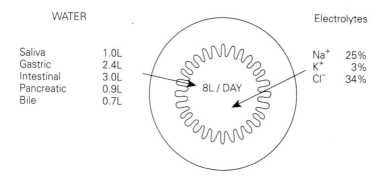

Fig. 4.2 Daily water and electrolyte secretions of gastro intestinal tract. Approximately 20% (eight litres) of total body water is secreted into the digestive tract each day. The values given for electrolytes represent the percentage of total exchangeable electrolyte in the body. 25% of the total body exchangeable Na^+ is secreted into the gut each day. Three per cent of total body exchangeable K^+ represents 30% of the total extracellular fluid K^+. Normally, almost all of the water and electrolytes would be reabsorbed from the gut but with diarrhoea significant water and electrolyte loss can occur in the stool.

has potential to severely disrupt body water and electrolyte balance and create severe hypovolaemia as well as disturbances in acid base balance.

Diarrhoea is associated with loss of isosmotic fluid which causes hypovolaemia but does not directly alter plasma osmolarity or plasma Na^+ concentration. Even though plasma osmolarity may be normal diarrhoea causes thirst and renal Na^+ and water retention due to the effects of hypovolaemia on the renal and cardiac volume receptors.

Free water clearance

Normal plasma osmolarity is regulated within a relatively narrow range (280–290 mosmol/litre) despite periodic intake of water and solute. Regulation of plasma osmolarity involves excretion or retention of water when the kidney produces urine which is either hyperosmotic or hypoosmotic to plasma. The amount of water which is reabsorbed or excreted is often referred to as *free water clearance*. This is a confusing term and it is unfortunate that it is often used in the clinical literature. Free water clearance is not really a true clearance value but it refers to the volume of pure water (water free of solute) that would need to be removed or added to the urine to make it isosmotic with plasma.The term can perhaps be better understood by considering how the renal tubule handles water.

The ultrafiltrate of plasma which enters the renal tubule at the glomerulus has the same osmolarity as plasma and if this fluid was lost unchanged in the urine there would be no immediate change in plasma osmolarity and no loss or gain of free water, although there would be a decrease in extracellular fluid volume. The loop of Henle can be considered as generating free water by NaCl reabsorption without water, so that the renal tubular fluid, by the time it leaves the ascending limb of the loop of Henle, is made hypotonic to plasma. The hypotonic fluid leaving the loop of Henle is usually modified by water reabsorption across the medullary collecting tubules and the permeability of these tubules to water is regulated by ADH secretion.

The clearance of free water is zero if the urine is isosmotic to plasma and is positive when the urine is hypoosmotic to plasma, and negative when the urine is hyperosmotic to plasma. Negative free water clearance is a cumbersome term which refers to the amount of free water reabsorbed from the renal tubule, or to the amount of water that would have to be added to urine to make it isotonic to plasma.

In humans on a normal diet the maximum volume of free water that can be reabsorbed each day is around 2–2.5 litre, which does not seem a lot compared to the 10–20 litre of free water which can be excreted each day. However, changes in the osmolarity of plasma are not only defended by free water reabsorption as this would normally be supplemented by an increased water intake. The combined mechanisms of free water reabsorption and increased water intake effectively contol any tendency

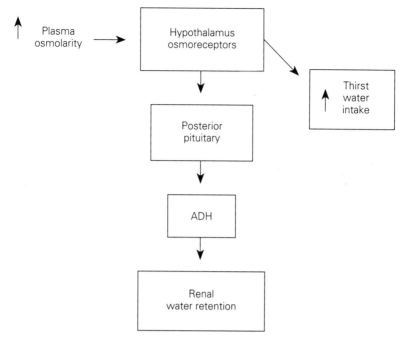

Fig. 4.3   Regulation of plasma osmolarity. An increase in plasma osmolarity stimulates hypothalamic osmoreceptors and causes ADH release from the pituitary and a sensation of thirst. ADH causes renal water retention and thirst increases water intake. Both these responses tend to return plasma osmolarity back towards normal.

for plasma osmolarity to rise above the normal range and the great capacity for free water excretion protects against any fall in plasma osmolarity.

Regulation of plasma osmolarity

The osmoreceptors in the hypothalamus sense plasma osmolarity and regulate thirst and ADH secretion as illustrated in Fig. 4.3. ADH is an octapeptide which is synthesised in the supraoptic and paraventricular nuclei of the hypothalamus and stored and secreted by the posterior pituitary. An increase in plasma osmolarity, for example due to dehydration, stimulates hypothalamic osmoreceptors which cause ADH release and thirst. The osmoreceptors that control thirst and those that control ADH release are not identical but are located close to each other in the wall of the third ventricle. The osmoreceptors do not respond to ineffective osmoles such as urea, alcohol and glucose but do respond to changes in effective osmoles such as Na^+. In the conscious person thirst will lead to increased water intake which will tend to restore body water balance and plasma osmolarity. The osmotic threshold for thirst is considerably higher than the osmotic threshold for ADH secretion and renal water conservation via ADH is maximal before thirst is perceived. Thirst is often associated with extracellular fluid volume depletion and in this case thirst is due to the effects of angiotensin II on the hypothalamic thirst mechanism. Hypovolaeima also leads to an increase in ADH release via the arterial barroreceptor reflex and cardiac atrial reflexes.

ADH acts on the renal collecting tubules causing an increase in permeability to water and water retention. In the presence of ADH a hyperosmotic urine is formed and obligatory solute loss occurs with a small volume of concentrated urine.

With a decrease in plasma osmolarity due to excessive water intake, thirst is inhibited and ADH secretion is inhibited by the hypothalamic osmoreceptors. In the absence of ADH a large volume of hypoosmotic urine is formed and excess water is readily excreted. Up to 10 litres/day of water can be readily excreted by normal kidneys. Water intoxication and hypoosmolarity of plasma only occur when the water load is so great that the minimum osmolarity of the urine is reached. For example, if the daily solute load excreted by the kidney was 800 mosmol and the kidneys could produce urine at a minimum osmolarity of 80 mosmol, then only a maximum of 10 litres of urine could be formed. Any water intake in excess of this maximum urine volume would be retained and cause hypoosmolarity of the plasma. With a maximum urine volume of 10 litres it would be difficult to exceed this maximum by simple ingestion of water, however, when renal function is disturbed the ability of the kidneys to form dilute urine is affected and plasma hypoosmolarity may then be caused by normal water intake.

In normal healthy subjects with free access to water the volume of urine is determined by water intake and its effect on ADH secretion. In this condition there is usually an excess of water over that required as a solvent for obligatory loss of solutes such as urea and electrolytes. The osmolarity of urine in health varies widely according to the amounts of solute and water to be excreted and these are obviously related to diet and drinking habits.

Summary

Plasma osmolarity is regulated within a narrow range by balancing water intake and loss. The osmoreceptors of the hypothalamus sense plasma osmolarity and regulate the thirst mechanism and ADH secretion. Plasma osmolarity is primarily determined by ADH secretion which regulates renal loss of water in the urine.

5 Disorders of osmolarity, hyponatraemia and hypernatraemia

The osmolarity of the extracellular fluid environment is controlled by regulation of water intake and loss. The simple diagram illustrated in Fig. 5.1

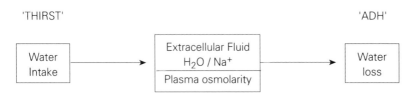

'THIRST'   'ADH'

Water Intake → Extracellular Fluid H₂O / Na⁺ / Plasma osmolarity → Water loss

Fig. 5.1 Control of plasma osmolarity. Plasma osmolarity is defended by two mechanisms. Thirst which regulates water intake and ADH secretion which regulates renal water loss.

should be kept in mind when discussing disturbances of osmolarity and plasma [Na⁺]. Plasma osmolarity is defended by two mechanisms, thirst and ADH secretion, and a disturbance in one mechanism can usually be compensated by changes in the other mechanism. So, for example, excessive water intake can be balanced by increased renal water loss under the influence of ADH without any clinically significant change in plasma osmolarity and plasma [Na⁺]. Similarly, excessive loss of water due to a disturbance in the secretion of ADH can be compensated by an increased intake of water, again without any clinically significant change in plasma osmolarity and plasma [Na⁺].

A change in plasma [Na⁺] has no direct physiological effects except those related to changes in plasma osmolarity. Since cell membranes are relatively impermeable to Na⁺ changes in extracellular fluid [Na⁺] have little effect on the resting membrane potential. This is in contrast, for example, with changes in extracellular [K⁺] which readily change the resting membrane potential in cardiac tissue. The symptoms related to changes in plasma [Na⁺] are therefore caused by changes in plasma osmolarity which may cause cells to expand or shrink. These changes in cell volume mainly affect the brain and result in a wide range of non-specific symptoms varying from headache and lethargy up to coma and convulsions. A slow change in plasma [Na$^+$] is usually well tolerated and may result in an abnormal plasma [Na$^+$] with few related symptoms. In contrast an acute change in plasma [Na$^+$] can rapidly result in coma, convulsions and death.

Disturbances in plasma [Na$^+$] and plasma osmolarity are often diagnosed from a routine blood electrolyte request and are therefore a laboratory diagnosis rather than a clinical diagnosis based on signs and symptoms.

Disorders of water balance

Disorders of water intake and loss are listed in Fig. 5.2. A decreased water intake below normal requirements is rare in the conscious patient with free access to water as water intake is governed by thirst. In the unconscious patient and infant water deprivation may inadvertently occur and result in clinically significant changes in osmolarity and plasma [Na$^+$]. Excessive loss of water from the body may be due to failure of ADH secretion or failure of the kidneys to respond to ADH these conditions result in a copious flow of very dilute urine (diabetes insipidus). Central diabetes insipidus is caused by decreased secretion of ADH and nephrogenic diabetes insipidus by a failure of the kidney to respond to ADH. Central diabetes insipidus is often caused by head trauma whereas nephrogenic diabetes insipidus is related to hypercalcemia, hypokalaemia and osmotic diuresis.

Patients with excessive water loss due to central or nephrogenic diabetes insipidus complain of polydipsia and polyuria rather than symptoms related to hypernatraemia. Plasma [Na$^+$] may be kept close to normal because a great increase in water intake occurs due to thirst, and this matches the water loss in the urine. Central and nephrogenic diabetes insipidus result in polyuria with a large volume of dilute urine and this is the main clinical sign. The increase in plasma osmolarity associated with these conditions is sufficent to activate the thirst mechanism but is not usually great enough to elicit other symptoms related to dehydration and hypernatraemia. Dipsogenic diabetes insipidus due to excessive intake of water is also associated with polyuria but here there is a decrease in plasma osmolarity due to dilution of body fluids. Any change in plasma osmolarity due to excessive water intake is limited by increased water loss, and symptoms related to brain oedema and hyponatraemia do not usually occur.

Although in theory it should be easy to differentiate between the different causes of polyuria in practice there is much overlap of plasma osmolarity values which makes differential diagnosis difficult. In theory those patients with central and nephrogenic diabetes insipidus should have a high plasma osmolarity and those with dipsogenic diabetes insipidus a low plasma osmolarity, but in practice, thirst and renal excretion of water tend to prevent major changes in osmolarity and blur the distinction between the groups. Clinical history is probably just as useful as laboratory tests as

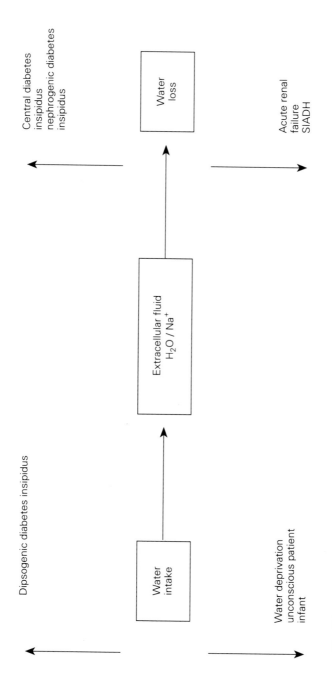

Fig. 5.2 Disorders of water balance are caused by either a change in water intake or a change in water loss.

the results from water deprivation tests and even plasma levels of ADH are often open to criticism.

Disorders of water balance due to low levels of secretion of ADH (central diabetes insipidus) can be treated by administration of either ADH or ADH analogues. ADH treatment needs to be carefully monitored in patients with heart disease, as ADH or vasopressin as it is sometimes named can cause arteriolar vasoconstriction and myocardial ischaemia. The vasoconstrictor activity of ADH is also used for the treatment of bleeding oesophageal varices as ADH causes splanchnic vasoconstriction and reduces portal venous pressure.

Hyponatraemia and hypoosmolar states

Na^+ is the major osmole of plasma and as previously discussed in Chapter 1, a good measure of plasma osmolarity is twice the plasma $[Na^+]$. Plasma osmolarity and plasma $[Na^+]$ are therefore directly related and a measurement of plasma osmolarity can often help to confirm a diagnosis of hyponatraemia or hypernatraemia.

The hypothalamic osmoreceptors are the guardian of plasma osmolarity and normally any reduction in plasma $[Na^+]$ accompanied by a reduction in plasma osmolarity would result in almost complete suppression of ADH secretion and subsequent diuresis. The excretion of a dilute urine would then rapidly return plasma $[Na^+]$ towards normal values. Therefore any condition of persistent hyponatraemia needs an explanation on the basis of why an increase in water excretion has not occurred or not been sufficient to return plasma $[Na^+]$ towards normal.

The development of hyponatraemia can be discussed in terms of two basic mechanisms either an increase in extracellular water which dilutes the plasma solutes or a loss of Na^+ which would have the same effect. Factors which can influence these two basic mechanisms are listed in Fig. 5.3. Excessive water intake beyond normal requirements will tend to dilute the extracellular fluid but with normal renal function a large volume of dilute urine will be formed and there will be no tendency for water to accumulate in the extracellular fluid compartment and little change in plasma osmolarity and plasma $[Na^+]$. However if there is some change in the ability of the renal system to excrete water, for example due to acute renal failure or inappropriate secretion of ADH, then water will accumulate in the extracellular compartment and the resulting hypoosmolarity and hyponatraemia may be sufficient to cause non-specific symptoms related to brain oedema.

Redistribution of Na^+ and water between the intracellular and extracellular compartments can also cause hyponatraemia without any change in the absolute amounts of Na^+ and water. Hyponatraemia may be caused by infusion of solutes such as mannitol or glucose which cause an increase in plasma osmolarity and an acute movement of water to the extracellular compartment. In this condition the hyponatraemia is associated with an

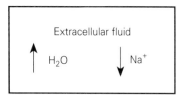

- Excessive water intake
- Decreased ability of kidney to excrete water
- Movement of water from intracellular to extracellular compartment

- Na^+ loss via kidney gut and skin
- Movement of Na^+ from extracellular to intracellular compartment

Fig. 5.3 Causes of hyponatremia. The figure lists the factors associated with an increase in total body water and a decrease in total exchangeable Na^+.

increase in plasma osmolarity due to the presence of the inflused solutes. The acute hyponatraemia caused by mannitol infusion can subsequently change to hypernatraemia as the osmotic action of mannitol causes renal water loss due to an osmotic diuresis.

Movement of Na^+ from the extracellular compartment to the intracellular compartment will also cause dilution of extracellular fluid and this shift can occur as a result of K^+ depletion. With K^+ depletion Na^+ and H^+ move into the intracellular compartment in order to maintain electrical neutrality.

Hyponatraemia is more commonly related to water imbalance rather than Na^+ loss but in some instances loss of Na^+ via the kidney, gut and skin can cause hyponatraemia, especially if the electrolyte loss is associated with hypovolaemia.

Clinical causes for hyponatraemia

The normal plasma $[Na^+]$ is around 145 meq/litre and a plasma $[Na^+]$ below 135 meq/litre is usually described as hyponatraemia. This level of hyponatraemia is usually associated with hypoosmolarity. The most common causes of hyponatraemia are listed in Table 5.1.

Diuretics

Diuretic treatment often results in a mild hyponatraemia which is not usually of clinical significance unless there are other complications. Excessive diuretic therapy may cause hyponatraemia via three mechanisms; due to

Table 5.1   Causes of hyponatremia

Diuretic therapy
Hypovolaemia
Cardiac failure
Syndrome of inappropriate ADH (SIADH)
Acute renal failure

hypovolaemia; K^+ depletion and due to direct inhibition of urinary dilution by diminished NaCl reabsorption in the diluting segments of the kidney.

Hypovolaemia

Hypovolaemia due to vomiting, diarrhoea and renal water loss is often associated with hyponatraemia. The hypovolaemia in these cases is associated with both water and solute loss and the mechanism is illustrated in Fig. 5.4. Water loss is readily replaced by drinking but this will result in plasma dilution. Normally the dilution of plasma would be limited by renal excretion of water, but hypovolaemia stimulates ADH release and thirst via the barroreceptor reflex and atrial reflexes. Hypovolaemia will also stimulate formation of angiotensin which is a potent stimulus to thirst. The angiotensin-aldosterone system will also promote renal conservation of Na^+ but this will only be effective in the long term and cannot balance an acute loss of solute. Hypovolaemia also causes hyponatraemia and hypoosmolarity by decreasing renal perfusion and the delivery of water to

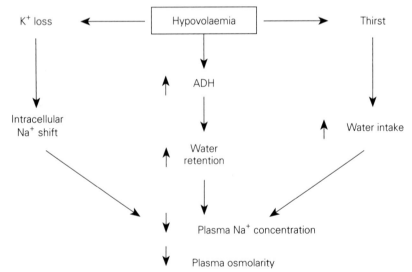

Fig. 5.4   Hyponatremia caused by hypovolaemia. Hypovolaemia due to vomiting, diarrhoea and renal losses can cause hyponatremia due to increased water retention, K^+ loss and increased water intake.

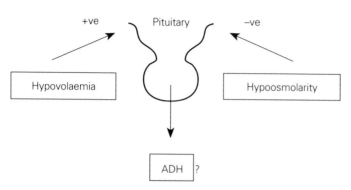

Fig. 5.5   Hypovolaemia associated with plasma hypoosmolarity causes a conflict of signals as regards the secretion of ADH. In this situation the signal related to hypovolaemia takes priority and ADH secretion causes water retention.

the diluting segments of the kidney, thus limiting water excretion. Diarrhoea and vomiting which are common causes of hypovolaemia are often associated with K^+ depletion which causes an intracellular movement of Na^+ and H^+ and acts as another mechanism leading towards hyponatraemia.

The combination of hypovolaemia and hypoosmolarity present conflicting signals to the control mechanism for ADH release as shown in Fig. 5.5. The signals from the arterial barroreceptos and atrial receptors indicate hypovolaemia and stimulate ADH release, whereas the plasma hypoosmolarity inhibits ADH release via the hypothalamic osmoreceptors. In this conflict situation between hypovolaemia and hypoosmolarity it is hypovolaemia that take precedence and water retention occurs in response to increased ADH secretion.

Cardiac failure

Hyponatraemia can also be associated with conditions that cause an increase in extracellular fluid volume. Cardiac failure can result in hyponatraemia with increased extracellular fluid volume and here a fall in arterial blood pressure stimulates ADH release via the barroreceptor reflex. Increased levels of ADH lead to water retention and this response may be exaggerated if the ability of the kidney to excrete water is compromised by a fall in renal perfusion. Congestive cardiac failure is associated with increased blood levels of atrial natriuretic factor and since this promotes renal loss of Na^+ this is a contributing factor in the development of hyponatraemia.

Syndrome of inappropriate ADH (SIADH)

Changes in plasma [Na^+] are usually secondary to a change in total body water and therefore it is not surprising that disturbances in ADH secretion cause hyponatraemia. Inappropriate ADH secretion is often termed syndrome of inappropriate ADH (SIADH). In SIADH, ADH secretion is unrelated to extracellular fluid volume or osmolarity. SIADH may be related to various causes: brain damage affecting hypothalamic control or pituitary secretion of ADH; ectopic ADH from oat cell carcinoma of lung; postoperative recovery; and treatment with the oral hypoglycemic drug chlorpropamide which potentiates the effects of ADH. SIADH is associated with high levels of ADH and water retention. Oedema does not occur as the increase in extracellular fluid volume causes inhibition of aldosterone release and an increased urinary Na^+ loss.

Hyponatraemia due to SIADH is caused by both water retention and Na^+ loss. Ingestion of water is an important factor in the development of hyponatraemia in SIADH as if water intake is restricted water retention and Na^+ loss do not occur and hyponatraemia does not develop.

Sick cell syndrome

In severely ill patients hyponatraemia may occur due to a widespread increase in cell permeability and intracellular movement of Na^+. The hyponatraemia improves and worsens according to the condition of the patient. This condition is often termed 'sick cell syndrome' and may occur in the severely ill post-surgical patient. The cause of the condition is unknown but appears to be related to a breakdown in cell metabolism due to poor circulation, hypoxia and endocrine disturbances which disturb the active transport of Na^+ and K^+ across the cell membrane. The hyponatraemia may respond to any measures that support the functions of the cardiovascular and respiratory systems and to insulin and glucose infusion. These measures are believed to restore cell metabolism and promote the activity of the Na^+/K^+ pump across the cell membrane.

Acute renal failure

In acute renal failure the ability of the kidney to form urine is reduced and both water and salt retention occur. Water is usually retained in excess of salt and this often results in hyponatraemia.

Pseudohyponatraemia

A false hyponatraemia or pseudohyponatraemia may be caused by hyperlipidaemia and hyperproteinaemia. The concentration of Na^+ in the plasma water is normal but there is an apparent dilution of the plasma [Na^+] due to abnormally high amounts of lipid or protein. There are no symptoms related to pseudohyponatraemia as the [Na$^+$] in the extracellular water is normal.

Diagnosis of hyponatraemia

Pseudohyponatraemia should first be excluded by determination of plasma lipid and protein levels. A low plasma [Na$^+$] and normal osmolarity in the absence of hyperglycemia and azotemia strongly suggests pseudohyponatremia. Hyponatraemia is not always accompanied by plasma hypoosmolarity as other solutes such as ethanol and mannitol may compensate for a low plasma [Na$^+$]. Hyponatraemia may result from excessive water intake or inadequate renal excretion of water. A history of polydipsia and excretion of large volumes of dilute urine is an obvious diagnosis for excessive water intake (dipsogenic diabetes insipidus) but this is a relatively uncommon cause of hyponatraemia. A mild hyponatraemia is often associated with diuretic therapy but clinically significant hyponatraemia is more commonly caused by impaired renal excretion of water and this may be due to one of three mechanisms; acute renal failure, inappropriate secretion of ADH and a slow flow of urine through the collecting ducts due to renal vascular disease and congestive heart failure.

Treatment of hyponatraemia

Treatment of hyponatraemia should never be started solely on the basis of laboratory findings as the diagnosis and treatment depend on a careful assessment of the clinical history. Acute severe hyponatraemia can be life threatening due to brain oedema but over-rapid correction of hyponatraemia can also be dangerous due to volume overload and brain dehydration. Clinical opinion is divided concerning the benefits and dangers of rapid correction of hyponatraemia but in general the speed of correction should be related to the duration of hyponatraemia with rapid correction reserved for an acute history with life-threatening symptoms. Rapid correction of plasma [Na$^+$] can be achieved by removal of excess body water with a loop diuretic such as furosemide together with administration of hypertonic saline. Slow correction of hyponatraemia can often be achieved with water restriction alone and if this is unsuccessful treatment with a loop diuretic and increased intake of salt and potassium may be tried. Hyponatraemia associated with hypovolaemia can usually be treated with intravenous infusion of normal saline and hyponatraemia in normovolaemic patients, oedematous patients, and those with SIADH can often be treated by restricting water intake together with treatment of any underlying disease responsible for the electrolyte disturbance.

Hypernatraemia and hyperosmolar states

Hypernatraemia results in plasma hyperosmolarity since the major osmole of the plasma is Na^+. A plasma $[Na^+]$ greater than 150 meq/litre can be defined as hypernatraemia. An acute increase in plasma $[Na^+]$ up to 158 meq/litre can cause neurological symptoms but chronic hyponatraemia may be without symptoms even with plasma $[Na^+]$ as high as 170 meq/litre. For each milliequivalent increase in $[Na^+]$ the plasma osmolarity will increase by two milliosmoles as Na^+ is accompanied by an anion.

Hypernatraemia is caused by excessive water loss or Na^+ retention. Excessive water loss is the most common cause of hypernatraemia particularly in infants or comatose patients who cannot voluntarily increase water intake. Hyperosmolarity stimulates ADH release and thirst. The thirst mechanism and water ingestion are the main factors which protect against hypernatraemia and hyperosmolarity as water retention by the kidney is only effective following water intake. In the unconscious patient the thirst mechanism is obviously inoperative and it is here that there is a danger of severe hypernatraemia.

An increase in plasma osmolarity causes water movement out of cells and brain dehydration which results in neurologic symptoms such as lethargy, weakness, twitching, seizures and eventual coma.

Thirst is very effective at increasing water intake and hypernatraemia is not usually severe in an alert patient with access to water.

The kidney has a great capacity to excrete excess NaCl if there is adequate water intake and therefore hypernatraemia due to excessive ingestion of NaCl or therapeutic error with administration of NaCl is not so common. Increased water loss can occur with sweating, burns and renal loss due to diabetes insipidus of central or renal origin. Loss of secretions from the digestive tract due to vomiting or diarrhoea does not cause hypernatraemia as the secretions are isosmotic with plasma and the resulting hypovolaemia stimulates water retention and can lead to hyponatraemia.

Fluid lost from sweating and the respiratory tract is hypoosmotic to plasma and fever and respiratory infections can lead to hypernatraemia, particularly in infants and comatose patients who cannot increase water intake.

Treatment of hypernatraemia involves administration of water as it is only rarely that the hypernatraemia is due to excess solute. Rapid correction of hypernatraemia can be lethal as brain oedema may result if water enters the cells too quickly. Hypotonic NaCl solution slowly infused with serial measurements of plasma $[Na^+]$ can be prescribed until the plasma $[Na^+]$ returns towards normal.

Summary

Hyponatraemia and hypernatraemia are disorders of water balance rather than Na^+ balance. Hyponatraemia is caused by water retention in excess of body solute whereas hypernatraemia is caused by excessive water loss. ADH plays a central role in the disorders and most conditions can be related to a disturbance in the renal handling of water.

6   Acid base balance

An acid is defined as a substance that can donate hydrogen ions and a base as a substance that can accept hydrogen ions. An acid such as carbonic acid dissociates to give a hydrogen ion H^+ and a bicarbonate ion HCO_3^-. The bicarbonate is a base as it can accept hydrogen ions to reform the carbonic acid.

The regulation of the concentration of hydrogen ions within and around the cells of the body is vital for survival. All of the proteins of the body are influenced by hydrogen ion concentration and the rate of any enzymatic reaction can be disrupted by changes in hydrogen ion concentration. The plasma concentration of hydrogen ions affects the distribution and state of ionisation of electrolytes such as potassium and calcium, and disturbances in hydrogen ion concentration can cause serious electrolyte disorders.

The first and most important point to note about hydrogen ions is that it is the free hydrogen ion in solution that influences biological activity. When we measure the concentration of free hydrogen ions in solution we are dealing with tiny amounts compared to the concentrations of say bicarbonate or potassium ions or any other plasma electrolyte. For example, in normal plasma the concentration of electrolytes is measured in *milli equivalents* with plasma $[Na^+]$ at 142 meq/litre and plasma $[HCO_3^-]$ at 24 meq/litre. Hydrogen ion concentration is measured in units a million times smaller *nano equivalents* with plasma $[H^+]$ normally around 40 nano eq/litre (0.00004 meq/litre). Therefore in normal plasma there are around three and a half million bicarbonate ions to each free hydrogen ion.

Instead of discussing $[H^+]$ in terms of nanoequivalents the pH scale is normally used with normal blood $[H^+]$ equal to pH 7.4

$$pH = \log \frac{1}{[H^+]}$$

The pH measures only the concentration of free H^+, and H^+ buffered on haemoglobin or phosphates, etc., is not included. Buffering of H^+ effectively stabilises the $[H^+]$, and the buffer systems within the body have an extremely important role in controlling the $[H^+]$ around cells.

Sources of H^+

Acids and alkalis can be taken in with the diet but this is only a minor

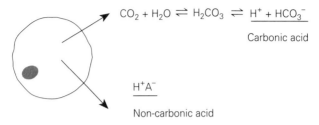

$$CO_2 + H_2O \rightleftharpoons H_2CO_3 \rightleftharpoons \underline{H^+ + HCO_3^-}$$

Carbonic acid

$$\underline{H^+A^-}$$

Non-carbonic acid

Fig. 6.1   Sources of acid from cellular metabolism. 15 moles of CO_2 (carbonic acid) and 50–100 meq of non-carbonic acids are produced each day.

source of acid base disturbance when compared to the very large amounts of H^+ generated by normal metabolic activity each day. There are two types of acid generated by metabolism, *carbonic acid* and other acids termed *non-carbonic acids*. Carbonic acid is formed from CO_2 and non-carbonic acids include mineral acids such as sulphuric acid and organic acids such as lactic acid. The separation of body acids into these two groups simplifies discussion as they are buffered in different ways by the body.

The generation of carbonic and non-carbonic acids is illustrated in Fig. 6.1. CO_2 is generated on oxidation of carbon, for example during normal oxidative metabolism of glucose. Non-carbonic acids are generated during metabolism of amino acids, for example sulphuric acid on oxidation of sulphur containing amino acids. Non-carbonic acids are also generated during anaerobic metabolism, e.g. lactic acid, and with metabolic disorders such as diabetes mellitus, e.g. acetoacetic acid.

Far much more carbonic acid is generated than non-carbonic acids. For example, 15 moles of CO_2 are produced each day and during the course of its transport to the lungs approximately three quarters of this is converted to carbonic acid. Therefore the body is dealing with (15.0 x 0.75) or 11 moles of carbonic acid each day. Each mole of CO_2 will form one equivalent of carbonic acid and thus 11 equivalents of carbonic acid are formed each day.

Compared to the production of 11 equivalents of carbonic acid the 50–100 meq of non-carbonic acids produced each day seems small but when this daily acid load is compared against the normal concentration of free H^+ in body fluids the daily production of non-carbonic acid is enormous. At pH 7.4 the concentration of free H^+ is 40 nano eq/litre (0.00004 meq/litre) and if for ease of calculation we say total body water equals 50 litre then free H^+ equally distributed throughout body water would only total (50 x 0.00004) or 0.002 meq.

This then nicely states the problem of handling acids in the body. Metabolism produces approximately 11 equivalents of carbonic acid and 50–100 meq of non-carbonic acid each day, and with buffering and excretion of H^+ the free H^+ concentration in blood is stabilised at 40 nano eq/litre (0.00004 meq/litre). The range of free H^+ compatible with life is from 16–160 nano eq/litre (pH 7.8–6.8).

To state the problem another way it is comparable to the body maintaining the plasma $[Na^+]$ at 142 meq/litre whilst at the same time over 500 kg of NaCl is ingested each day. Because of the very large amount of H^+ produced each day buffering of H^+ is of prime importance in limiting the free $[H^+]$ in plasma prior to excretion of the acids.

Buffering of H+

An acid consists of hydrogen ions H^+ and anions A^-. In a strong mineral acid such as hydrochloric acid nearly all of the H^+ is free and there is little undissociated acid HA. In a weak acid such as carbonic acid or lactic acid very few of the H^+ is free and there is much undissociated acid HA. In any acid there is an equilibrium between the undissociated acid HA and free H^+ as shown below.

$$HA \rightleftharpoons H^+ A^-$$

In a weak acid the equilibrium lies well over to the left with little free H^+ and much undissociated acid, HA.

A buffer solution consists of a weak acid which is mainly in the form of the undissociated acid HA and its salt which consists of the anion of the acid associated with a cation such as Na^+ or K^+.

For example, in the erythrocyte, haemoglobin is a weak acid and it also exists as a K^+ salt.

$$H\,Hb \rightleftharpoons H^+ + Hb^-$$
$$K\,Hb \rightleftharpoons K^+ + Hb^-$$

The buffering process involves formation of a weak undissociated acid so that the free H^+ generated by metabolism is bound to the anion of the weak acid (Hb^-).

In the erythrocyte haemoglobin buffers carbonic acid as follows:

$$H^+HCO_3^- + K^+Hb^- \rightleftharpoons H^+Hb^- + K^+HCO_3^-$$

The buffering of carbonic acid produced by metabolic activity in the tissues is also an important link for O_2 transport as the association of haemoglobin with H^+ during the buffering causes a decrease in the affinity of haemoglobin for O_2. The buffering process in the erythrocyte is illustrated in Fig. 6.2.

Carbonic and non-carbonic acids are handled in different ways in the body, they are buffered on different buffers and excreted by different mechanisms.

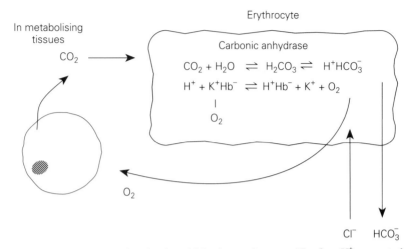

Fig. 6.2   Buffering of carbonic acid in the erythrocyte. The free H^+ generated with carbonic acid is buffered on the haemoglobin protein chain. The buffering of the H^+ decreases the affinity of haemoglobin for O_2 and aids in the delivery of O_2 to the tissues. HCO_3^- diffuses out of the erythrocyte down a concentration gradient and in order to maintain electrical neutrality Cl^- ions move into the erythrocyte. These reactions are reversed when the erythrocyte enters the lungs and haemoglobin is oxygenated.

Buffering and excretion of carbonic acid

As discussed above the metabolic activity of the body generates a very large amount of carbonic acid each day. If this acid were not removed from the body in the form of gaseous CO_2 the $[H^+]$ in the blood would very rapidly reach lethal levels. During its transport from the tissues to the lungs the carbonic acid is buffered on haemoglobin as shown in Fig. 6.2. Thus haemoglobin temporarily buffers the free H^+ from carbonic acid and therefore prevents any major change in blood $[H^+]$ associated with CO_2 production. However, it is necessary for the buffer to be renewed and the source of the H^+, namely the CO_2 excreted to prevent accumulation of acid. Excretion of CO_2 occurs in the lungs where CO_2 is expired to the atmosphere. Uptake of O_2 in the lungs oxygenates haemoglobin and this facilitates liberation of the H^+ and allows it to combine with HCO_3^- to regenerate CO_2. Oxygenated haemoglobin is a stronger acid than deoxygenated haemoglobin as it more readily releases the associated H^+. This change in the affinity of haemoglobin for H^+ is important in the buffering process.

In the tissues CO_2 is converted to carbonic acid in the erythrocyte and the free H^+ is buffered on haemoglobin. In the lungs the H^+ liberated from haemoglobin recombine with HCO_3^- to form carbonic acid which is then lost to the atmosphere as CO_2.

CO_2 is a waste product of metabolism but it also occupies a central position in the bodies defences against acid base disturbances as part of the carbonic acid-bicarbonate buffer system. The arterial level of dissolved CO_2 is closely regulated by the respiratory system at PCO_2 40 mm Hg or 5 kPa. This partial pressure of carbon dioxide is much greater than that in the atmosphere where there is only a trace present. Therefore the body retains carbonic acid at a regulated level in order to utilise the carbonic acid-bicarbonate buffer system as a defence against acid base disturbances. The role of this buffer system will be discussed later.

Buffering and excretion of non-carbonic acids

Non-carbonic acids consist of organic and mineral acid. Unlike carbonic acid they do not have a gaseous form and are therefore excreted via the kidneys rather than the lungs. The daily production of non-carbonic acids (such as sulphuric, lactic acid, etc.) is 50–100 meq but in diabetic keto acidosis this can be raised to over 500 meq a day.

The H^+ released by non-carbonic acids are buffered with HCO_3^-. The interstitial fluid around cells contains HCO_3^- and therefore the free H^+ of the acid is almost immediately neutralised as shown in Fig. 6.3. HCO_3^- is consumed during the buffering process and any increase in non-carbonic acid production such as with diabetic keto acidosis is associated with a fall in plasma $[HCO_3^-]$. The CO_2 generated on neutralisation of the acid is lost via respiration. Generation of CO_2 does not cause any disturbance in the blood levels of CO_2 as the amount generated by this reaction is insignificant compared to the very large amounts produced by normal cellular metabolism.

The sodium salt of the acid (Na^+A^-) is transported in the blood and filtered by the kidneys into the renal tubule. The renal tubule completes the excretion of the acid and regenerates HCO_3^- as illustrated in Fig. 6.4. Excretion of the H^+ is accomplished by the following processes:

1. Secretion of H^+ into the renal tubule which then associate with the anion of the acid A^-. In effect the acid ($H^+ A^-$) is regenerated in the renal tubule. The H^+ is buffered on urinary buffers.
2. Regeneration of the HCO_3^- which was originally consumed in the buffering process. The renal tubule reabsorbs HCO_3^- back into the plasma.
3. Retention of Na^+. The Na^+ which accompanied the anion of the acid A^- is not lost in the urine as this would strain the economy of Na^+ balance. Instead most of the Na^+ is reabsorbed by the renal tubule.

The urinary buffers of ammonia, phosphate and HCO_3^- are very important in the urinary excretion of non-carbonic acids. The minimum pH of urine is pH 4.5–5.0 as this represents the maximum concentration gradient against which transport of H^+ can be sustained across the renal tubule. If

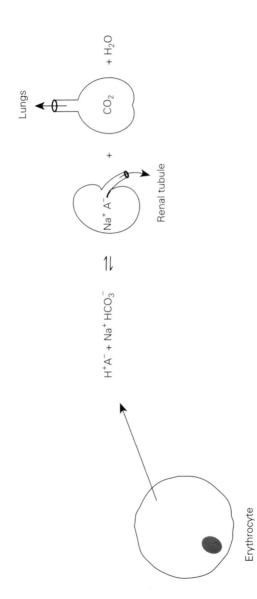

Fig. 6.3 Buffering of non-carbonic acids. HCO_3^- is consumed as the free H^+ of the acid is neutralised. The Na^+ salt of the acid $Na^+ A^-$ is filtered into the renal tubule to be handled by the kidney. The CO_2 produced by the reaction is lost via the respiratory system.

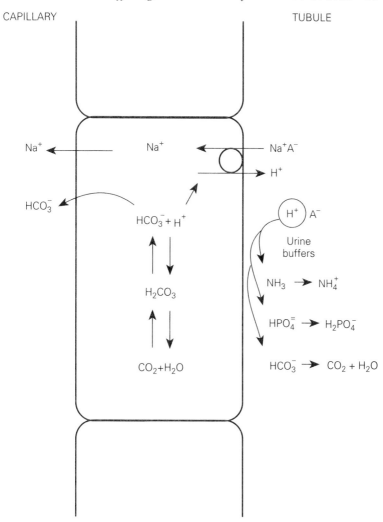

Fig. 6.4 Excretion of non-carbonic acid in the renal tubule. H$^+$ secreted by the renal tubule is exchanged for Na$^+$. The H$^+$ is buffered on ammonia, phosphate and HCO$_3^-$. HCO$_3^-$ generated by the renal tubule replaces the HCO$_3^-$ originally consumed in the buffering of the acid.

we estimate the daily urine volume as 1.5 litre then 1.5 litre of urine at pH 4.5 contains only 0.05 meq of free H$^+$. Therefore without the urinary buffers the urine volume required to excrete a daily acid load of 100 meq H$^+$ would be in excess of 3000 litre.

In metabolic acidosis where the daily load of non-carbonic acids delivered to the kidney is greatly increased, the renal tubular production of ammonia is stimulated. Therefore the buffering capacity of the urine is increased to accommodate for the increased delivery of acid.

Special significance of carbonic acid–bicarbonate buffering system

The carbonic acid–bicarbonate buffering system is the main buffer system which controls blood pH. There are many buffer systems in the body, haemoglobin, phosphates, plasma proteins, etc., and they are important in limiting blood pH changes. However, unlike the carbonic acid–bicarbonate system they cannot be regulated in response to blood pH changes.

The pH of a buffer system is determined by the relative concentrations of the weak acid and its anion and this is expressed in the Henderson–Hasselbalch equation:

$$pH = pK + \log \frac{[A^-]}{[HA]}$$

where pK is a constant for any given system.

In the carbonic acid-bicarbonate system

$$pH = pK + \log \frac{[HCO_3^-]}{[H_2CO_3]}$$

The concentration of carbonic acid $[H_2CO_3]$ is directly related to the partial pressure of CO_2 and therefore for H_2CO_3 one can substitute PCO_2 x solubility constant therefore

$$pH = pK + \log \frac{[HCO_3^-]}{PCO_2 \text{ x } 0.0.3}$$

The pH of the buffer system is determined by the plasma $[HCO_3^-]$ concentration and PCO_2.

$$pH - \text{determined by} \frac{[HCO_3^-] \text{ (regulated by renal system)}}{PCO_2 \text{ (regulated by respiratory system)}}$$

The plasma $[HCO_3^-]$ is closely regulated by the renal system so that fluctuations above or below 24 meq/litre cause excretion or retention of HCO_3^-. The arterial PCO_2 is controlled by the respiratory system and fluctuations above or below PCO_2 40 mm Hg cause changes in ventilation which return the blood PCO_2 back towards normal.

With the plasma [HCO_3^-] fixed at 24 meq/litre and the arterial PCO_2 fixed at 40 mm Hg, the pH is fixed at pH 7.4 since pK is a fixed constant (6.1).

$$pH\ 7.4 = pK + \log \frac{[HCO_3^-\ 24\ meq/L]}{PCO_2\ 40\ mm\ Hg \times 0.03}$$

It is important to remember that it is the *ratio* of [HCO_3^-] to PCO_2 that determines the pH not the absolute values. So, for example, in metabolic acidosis the plasma [HCO_3^-] may be below normal and this causes an acidaemia. In order to compensate for this acidaemia ventilation is increased and this causes a fall in arterial PCO_2. Therefore the ratio of [HCO_3^-] to PCO_2 is brought closer to normal and the pH moves back towards pH 7.4 in the compensated condition even though both the plasma levels of [HCO_3^-] and PCO_2 are below normal.

All of the renal and respiratory compensatory responses which will be discussed later tend to bring the ratio of [HCO_3^-] and CO_2 back towards normal.

The body fluids contain several different buffer systems and one can consider this as a 'soup' of buffers. In such a mixture of buffers if the ratio of weak acid and anion of any one buffer system is fixed then this will determine the pH of the mixture and all other buffers will equilibrate around this pH. The renal and respiratory systems fix the concentrations of the weak acid and the anion of the carbonic acid–bicarbonate system and therefore fix the pH of all the buffer systems in the mixture at pH 7.4.

A unique property of the carbonic acid–bicarbonate buffer system is that the carbonic acid can easily be excreted in the form of CO_2. Therefore during buffering of a strong acid one of the end products can be removed.

$$H^+A^- + Na^+ HCO_3^- \rightleftharpoons H_2CO_3 + Na^+ A^- \rightleftharpoons H_2O + CO_2 + Na^+ A^-$$

Carbonic acid rapidly forms CO_2 and this can be lost via the respiratory system and this makes the buffer system much more effective. If CO_2 were not lost then addition of a strong acid would cause a much greater increase in free H^+.

The carbonic acid–bicarbonate buffer system is a very effective buffer for non-carbonic acids such as lactic acid and sulphuric acid but the HCO_3^- produced on hydration of CO_2 does not buffer the accompanying H^+.

$$CO_2 + H_2O \rightleftharpoons H_2CO_3 \rightleftharpoons H^+ + HCO_3^-$$

HCO_3^- is the anion of carbonic acid. Each H^+ that is generated on hydration of CO_2 is accompanied by HCO_3^-. This is completely different from the buffering of a non-carbonic acid such as hydrochloric acid where the buffering process consumes HCO_3^- and forms CO_2 The free H^+ generated by an increase in arterial PCO_2 is not buffered on HCO_3^- but is buffered on haemoglobin as previously described and to a much lesser extent on plasma proteins and phosphates.

One final point of significance about the carbonic acid–bicarbonate buffer system is that the concentration of carbonic acid can easily be determined by measuring plasma PCO_2 with a CO_2 electrode. The plasma pH is easily measured with a pH electrode and since two variables of the Henderson–Hasselbalch equation are then known (and pK is known to be a constant of 6.1) it is possible to calculate the third, the plasma $[HCO_3^-]$.

Because of the ease of measuring the components of the carbonic acid–bicarbonate system and because of its central role in controlling blood pH this buffer system is of especial clinical significance. The buffering properties of the carbonic acid–bicarbonate system are most easily understood when illustrated in the form of a pH - HCO_3^- graph

The pH/HCO_3^- graph

The carbonic acid–bicarbonate buffer system is described by the Henderson–Hasselbalch equation:

$$pH = pK + \log \frac{[HCO_3^-]}{[H_2CO_3] \text{ or } PCO_2 \times 0.03}$$

As mentioned above PCO_2 multiplied by a solubility constant (0.03) can be substituted for $[H_2CO_3]$. Like any equation the Henderson–Hasselbalch equation can be represented graphically, and in order to understand a graph of pH against HCO_3^- it is simpler to discuss an *in vitro* system before considering buffering in the patient. An *in vitro* system consisting of 1 litre of a solution of $NaHCO_3$ through which a mixture of air and CO_2 is bubbled to achieve a PCO_2 of 40 mm Hg is illustrated in Fig. 6.5. The pH, $[HCO_3^-]$ and PCO_2 within the solution can be plotted on a graph as shown in Fig. 6.6. Point A on the graph represents the conditions in the beaker with PCO_2 40 mm Hg, $[HCO_3^-]$ 24 meq/litre and pH 7.4. In this instance all three variables of the Henderson–Hasselbalch equation are known, but normally one would only need two values from the equation in order to calculate the third.

Buffering of non-carbonic acids

In order to illustrate graphically the buffering of a non-carbonic acid 12 meq of the strong mineral acid hydrochloric acid are added to the system and the results are shown in Fig. 6.7. The hydrochloric acid is buffered by the following reaction:

$$H^+Cl^- + Na^+ HCO_3^- \rightleftharpoons Na^+Cl^- + H_2O + CO_2$$

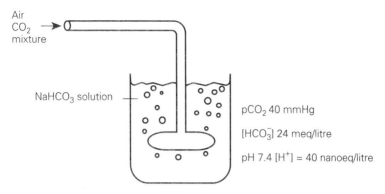

Fig. 6.5 *In vitro* system to demonstrate the properties of the pH/HCO$_3^-$ buffer system. The system consists of a beaker of Na HCO$_3$ solution continuously gassed with a mixture of CO$_2$ and air. The PCO$_2$ of the solution can be varied by changing the percentage of CO$_2$ in the gas mixture used for gassing.

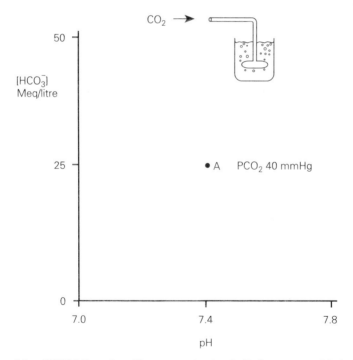

Fig. 6.6 pH/HCO$_3^-$ graph to illustrate an *in vitro* buffering system. CO$_2$ is bubbled through the NaHCO$_3$ solution to achieve a PCO$_2$ of 40 mmHg. With the [HCO$_3^-$] at 24 meq/litre the pH of the system is pH 7.4. These parameters are plotted on the pH/HCO$_3^-$ graph. Point A represents the conditions in the beaker at a PCO$_2$ of 40 mmHg.

some of the HCO_3^- in the solution is consumed during the buffering process as 12 meq of hydrochloric acid combine with 12 meq of HCO_3^- CO_2 is liberated and there is a transient rise in PCO_2 but this equilibrates at PCO_2 40 mm Hg as the system is an open system and not a closed bottle and the PCO_2 is determined by the rate of gassing. The buffer system is very effective as addition of 12 million nano eq of free H^+ to the beaker only causes the $[H^+]$ to rise from 40 nano eq/litre to 80 nano eq/litre and the pH changes from 7.4 to pH 7.1. The conditions achieved after addition of the hydrochloric acid are illustrated by point B in Fig. 6.7.

Although points A and B have different $[HCO_3^-]$ and pH values the PCO_2 is identical at PCO_2 40 mm Hg. All the points on the line joining A to B have the same PCO_2 40 mm Hg and this line is called an isobar PCO_2 40 mm Hg. Other isobars for PCO_2 60 mm Hg and PCO_2 20 mm Hg are

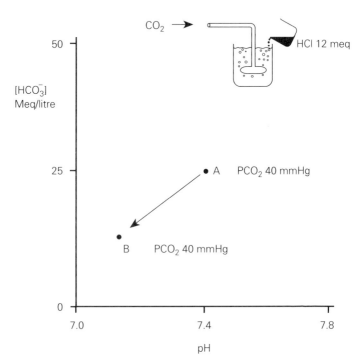

Fig. 6.7 pH/HCO_3^- graph to illustrate buffering of non-carbonic acid. Addition of a non carbonic acid such as hydrochloric acid to the buffer system in the beaker causes the acid to react with the HCO_3^- and the $[HCO_3^-]$ goes down as the $[H^+]$ concentration increases and pH decreases. Note, however, that in this open system there is no sustained increase in PCO_2 as any CO_2 generated by the buffering process is lost to the atmosphere and the PCO_2 is determined by the percentage of CO_2 in the gas mixture.

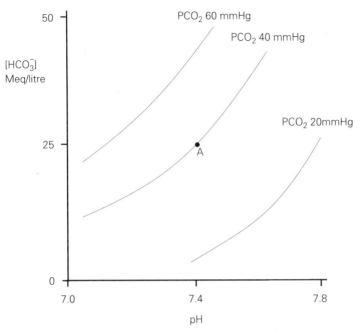

Fig. 6.8 pH/HCO₃⁻ graph to illustrate PCO₂ isobars. An isobar is a line linking all points with the same PCO₂. Point A is the normal point.

illustrated in Fig. 6.8. Any point on the pH–HCO₃ graph has a PCO_2 value as well as values for pH and [HCO₃⁻]. An isobar is a line linking all points with the same PCO_2 value.

Buffering of carbonic acid

The carbonic acid–bicarbonate buffer system in the beaker is a very effective buffer for non-carbonic acid but cannot buffer carbonic acid since the hydration of CO_2 generates HCO_3^-. The HCO_3^- solution in the beaker can be titrated with carbonic acid by changing the percentage of CO_2 in the gas mixture and thus altering the PCO_2 in the solution. The titration of a HCO_3^- solution with carbonic acid is illustrated in Fig. 6.9.

Carbonic acid is formed by the hydration of carbon dioxide as follows:

$$CO_2 + H_2O \rightleftharpoons H_2CO_3 \rightleftharpoons H^+ + HCO_3^-$$

The equilibrium lies well over to the left and there are approximately 340 molecules of CO_2 for each molecule of carbonic acid. However, an increase in PCO_2 does cause an increase in $[H^+]$ and decrease in pH as illustrated in Fig. 6.9. An increase in the PCO_2 in the solution causes an increase in the concentrations of carbonic acid and [HCO_3^-]. From the above equation it is apparent that for each H^+ generated a HCO_3^- is also generated. The line DAE in Fig. 6.9 illustrates the changes in pH and [HCO_3^-] brought about by changes in PCO_2. The change in pH from pH 7.0 to pH 7.8 represents a change in [H^+] from 100 to 16 nano eq/litre. The change in [HCO_3^-] will be of the same magnitude since each hydrogen ion generated from dissociation of carbonic acid is accompanied by HCO_3^-. However, the [HCO_3^-] in the Na HCO_3 solution in the beaker is around 25 meq/litre and the change in [HCO_3^-] caused by changes in gassing with CO_2 is only around 0.0001 meq/litre (100 nano eq/litre). The change in pH from 7.8 to 7.0 in Fig. 6.9 as one moves from point E to D represents uptake of only a tiny amount of CO_2 by the solution. The [HCO_3^-] is increased but the change is hardly measurable. Here one must also distinguish between PCO_2 and total CO_2 content. There is a great increase in PCO_2 from point E to D but the total CO_2 content of the solution has increased only very slightly with a little more dissolved CO_2 and a tiny increase in [HCO_3^-]. The total CO_2 content of a solution is defined as

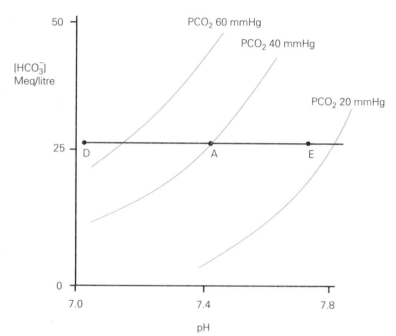

Fig. 6.9   pH/HCO_3^- graph to illustrate titration of $NaHCO_3$ solution with carbonic acid. An increase in the percentage of CO_2 in the gas mixture raises the PCO_2 in the solution and this is represented by point D. A decrease in the percentage of CO_2 in the gas mixture lowers the PCO_2 in the solution as represented by point E. Note that the [HCO_3^-] concentration increases as the PCO_2 rises due to formation of carbonic acid.

that amount of CO$_2$ which could be liberated from the solution on titration with a strong acid. In whole blood it therefore includes dissolved CO$_2$ and HCO$_3^-$ plus CO$_2$ bound to haemoglobin or plasma proteins.

The carbonic acid–bicarbonate buffer system can buffer non-carbonic acids very effectively, as described above, but it is not a buffer for carbonic acid.

Buffering of carbonic acid occurs on haemoglobin as haemoglobin accepts the hydrogen ion generated on dissociation of carbonic acid.

$$CO_2 + H_2O \rightleftharpoons H_2CO_3 \rightleftharpoons H^+ + HCO_3^-$$

$$\mid$$

Buffered on haemoglobin

The presence of haemoglobin as a buffer in blood means that most of the H$^+$ generated on hydration of CO$_2$ are buffered. CO$_2$ is hydrated in the erythrocyte to generate HCO$_3^-$ with only a limited rise in [H$^+$]. The hydration of CO$_2$ proceeds very slowly in aqueous solution but the presence of carbonic anhydrase in the erythrocyte accelerates the reaction so that it reaches equilibrium in a fraction of a second. The final equilibrium point for the reaction is not altered by carbonic anhydrase.

The buffering of carbonic acid in whole blood containing haemoglobin is compared with buffering in a Na HCO$_3$ solution in Fig. 6.10. The slope of the buffer line for whole blood is much steeper than that for Na HCO$_3$ solution and for any given change in PCO$_2$ the pH change is less in whole blood than that in the Na HCO$_3$ solution. The titration curve for whole blood is called the 'body buffer line'. The buffering of H$^+$ on haemoglobin means that whole blood when gassed with CO$_2$ has the capacity to absorb much more CO$_2$ than a similar solution of Na HCO$_3$.

A simple experiment illustrating the buffering properties of haemoglobin is demonstrated in Fig. 6.10. At point A the Na HCO$_3$ solution and blood have the same parameters as far as pH, PCO$_2$ and [HCO$_3^-$] are concerned. If the gassing with CO$_2$ through both solutions is now increased so that each achieves the same PCO$_2$ at 60 mm Hg then the blood will equilibrate with a higher [HCO$_3^-$] and lower [H$^+$] than the Na HCO$_3$ solution despite the fact the blood will have absorbed much more CO$_2$ than the Na HCO$_3$ solution. This result is apparent in Fig. 6.10 at points F and G on the PCO$_2$ 60 mm Hg isobar. The [HCO$_3^-$] at PCO$_2$ 60 mm Hg is much greater in blood than that in the Na HCO$_3$ solution because more CO$_2$ has been converted to carbonic acid. However the [H$^+$] is less in blood (pH greater) than in the NaHCO$_3$ solution because in blood each HCO$_3^-$ generated on dissociation of carbonic acid is not accompanied by a free H$^+$ as most are buffered on haemoglobin.

The buffering properties of plasma are similar to those of a Na HCO$_3$ solution as the plasma proteins have a much lower concentration than haemoglobin in blood. If one litre of whole blood and one litre of plasma are gassed with CO$_2$ to achieve the same PCO$_2$ the whole blood will

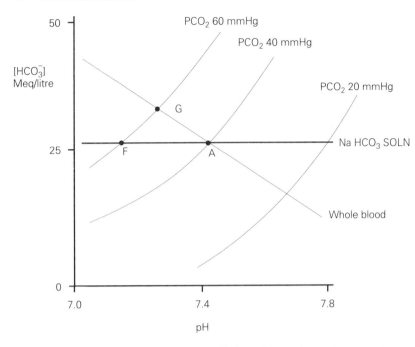

Fig. 6.10   pH/HCO$_3$⁻ graph to compare buffering of carbonic acid in whole blood with buffering in a Na HCO$_3$ solution. Titration of whole blood and a Na HCO$_3$ solution with CO$_2$ demonstrates that whole blood is a much more effective buffer than a Na HCO$_3$ solution. The haemoglobin in whole blood buffers the free H⁺ generated from carbonic acid.

absorb much more CO$_2$ and equilibrate with a higher [HCO$_3$⁻] and a lower [H⁺] concentration than the plasma. If the plasma and whole blood are now titrated with a strong acid to determine total CO$_2$ the blood will have a much greater total CO$_2$ content than the plasma.

Introduction to acid-base disturbances

The normal arterial blood pH 7.4 represents a free [H⁺] of only 40 nano eq/litre but the body produces 15 mol of CO$_2$ and 50–100 meq of non-carbonic acids each day. Therefore in acid base disturbances there is a great potential for this endogenous production of acid metabolites to cause a lethal increase in the blood [H⁺]. Similarly, loss of acid from the body associated with vomiting can cause an equally serious decrease in blood [H⁺]. Both acids and bases can cause disturbances in blood pH, but it is conventional to discuss these disturbances in terms of H⁺ balance as follows:

H^+ intake in food + H^+ production from metabolism

=

H^+ loss in urine + H^+ loss as CO_2 from lungs

As well as the above equation one also needs to consider the balance of acid and base in the gut as the gut recycles large amounts of acidic and alkaline secretions each day.

H^+ and HCO_3^- secretion into gut

=

H^+ and HCO_3^- reabsorbtion from gut

Acid base disturbances result when the equations do not balance, for example in diabetes mellitus when production of organic acids from metabolism exceeds the ability of the kidney to excrete them in the urine, or in vomiting or diarrhoea when acid or alkali are lost from the secretions of the gut and are therefore not available for reabsorption. Some common causes of acid base disturbance are listed in Table 7.3 (p. 95).

Acid base disturbances are normally described as *respiratory* or *metabolic*. These terms refer to the underlying disorder causing the acid base disturbance. In a respiratory disorder it is either depression or stimulation of ventilation that is the cause of the disorder. In a metabolic disorder the underlying condition may be related to excess H^+ production from metabolism, or disturbances of renal or gastro-intestinal function.

In the respiratory disorder, respiratory depression causes retention of CO_2 and this is referred to as *respiratory acidosis*. Whereas the loss of CO_2 caused by hyperventilation is referred to as *respiratory alkalosis*.

In the metabolic disorder, excess H^+ production from metabolism, decreased renal loss of H^+ or loss of HCO_3^- in diarrhoea are referred to as *metabolic acidosis*. Loss of acid with vomiting and renal loss of H^+ with diuretics and hyperaldosteronism are referred to as *metabolic alkalosis*.

The respiratory and metabolic disorders normally cause disturbances in blood pH as indicated by the terms acidosis and alkalosis.

However, in the compensated condition the respiratory or metabolic disorder may have a blood pH close to the normal pH 7.4. Mixed disorders may also occur so that an unconscious patient with metabolic acidosis who is hyperventilated on a respirator will have a PCO_2 lower than normal and this will result in a mixed metabolic acidosis/respiratory alkalosis and depending on the relative severity of each disorder the patients blood pH could be above or below pH 7.4.

Acidaemia refers to an arterial blood pH below pH 7.4 and *alkalaemia* to a blood pH greater than pH 7.4.

By convention it is normally arterial blood pH or extracellular pH that is implied in the terminology of acidosis/alkalosis, acidaemia/alkalaemia although strictly speaking one should consider both intracellular and extracellular pH as these may vary independently in metabolic but not respiratory disorders. Excessive K^+ loss, for example, which causes hypokalaemia can result in an intracellular acidosis with extracellular alkalosis.

Defence against acid base disturbance

The first lines of defence against acid base disturbance are the intracellular and extracellular buffers as these limit any change in $[H^+]$. Depending on the nature of the acid base disturbance there will then follow some compensatory change in respiratory and/or renal activity to restore the ratio of PCO_2 to $[HCO_3^-]$ concentration.

An increase in non-carbonic acid such as sulphuric acid or lactic acid is immediately buffered by reaction with HCO_3^- in interstitial fluid and blood. Over a period of hours H^+ enters the cellular compartment and is buffered on haemoglobin, phosphate and other intracellular buffers. The movement of H^+ into the cellular compartment displaces K^+ cations and this may lead to hyperkalaemia with a potentially serious elevation in plasma $[K^+]$. In the acute phase the non-carbonic acid is buffered with extracellular HCO_3^- but slow diffusion of H^+ intracellularly means that eventually up to 60% of the H^+ may be buffered intracellularly. Acidaemia associated with an increase in non-carbonic acid will stimulate renal and respiratory compensation as discussed later.

In contrast to non-carbonic acid almost all of the carbonic acid is buffered intracellularly, with haemoglobin playing a major role. CO_2 readily moves into the erythrocyte to form carbonic acid which dissociates to H^+ and HCO_3^- with the H^+ buffered on haemoglobin. If the acidaemia is severe and prolonged then H^+ may enter other cellular compartments such as bone. Since an increase in CO_2 and carbonic acid is caused by a respiratory disorder there can be no respiratory compensation but renal compensation will occur with increases in H^+ excretion and HCO_3^- reabsorption.

The causes and consequences of the respiratory and metabolic acid-base disturbances will be discussed in detail later.

Definition of acid base disturbance on pH/HCO$_3^-$ graph

Acid base disturbances can be defined on the pH/HCO$_3$ graph as illustrated in Fig. 6.11.

Respiratory disorders are defined according to the arterial PCO_2. If the PCO_2 is greater than PCO_2 40 mm Hg then the disorder has a component of respiratory acidosis and similarly if the PCO_2 is less than PCO_2 40 mmHg there is a component of respiratory alkalosis. On the pH/HCO$_3^-$ graph in Fig. 6.11 the respiratory disorders are classified as acidosis or alkalosis according to whether they lie to the left or right of the PCO_2 40 mmHg isobar. The metabolic disorders are classified as alkalosis or acidosis according to whether they lie above or below the body buffer line. The

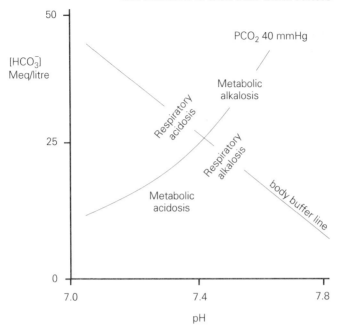

Fig. 6.11 Definition of acid base disturbances using the pH/HCO$_3^-$ graph. Acid base disturbances are defined according to the PCO$_2$ 40 mm Hg isobar and the body buffer line. All points to the left of the PCO$_2$ 40 mm Hg isobar have a component of respiratory acidosis and all points to the right of the isobar have a component of respiratory alkalosis. All points above the body buffer line have a component of metabolic alkalosis and all points below the body buffer line have a component of metabolic acidosis.

body buffer line represents the line obtained on titration of the blood sample with CO$_2$.

Metabolic disorders can also be defined according to the plasma [HCO$_3^-$] measured in a blood sample equilibrated at PCO$_2$ 40 mm Hg. If the plasma [HCO$_3^-$] in the blood is greater than 24 meq/litre at PCO$_2$ 40 mm Hg then there is a component of metabolic alkalosis and if the plasma [HCO$_3^-$] is less than 24 meq/litre at PCO$_2$ 40 mm Hg then there is a component of metabolic acidosis. When a sample of blood is drawn the PCO$_2$ may well be above or below PCO$_2$ 40 mm Hg but equilibration of the blood sample at PCO$_2$ 40 mm Hg eliminates any respiratory component that may also be present due to respiratory compensation and allows definition of any metabolic component. If when the blood sample is equilibrated at PCO$_2$ 40 mm Hg the plasma [HCO$_3^-$] is close to normal (24 meq/litre) then there is no metabolic component to the disorder and the disturbance may be due solely to a respiratory disorder. Some laboratories quote the plasma [HCO$_3^-$] measured at PCO$_2$ 40 mm Hg as *standard bicarbonate* and the deviation of $[HCO_3^-]$ above or below normal is quoted as *base excess* or *base deficit*.

Mixed disorders are common, for example the respiratory compensation of hyperventilation associated with metabolic acidosis causes a mixed metabolic acidosis/respiratory alkalosis. Renal compensation for a chronic respiratory acidosis causes a mixed respiratory acidosis/metabolic alkalosis.

The first step in diagnosing any acid base disturbance is to measure blood PCO_2, $[HCO_3^-]$ and pH. Plotting these parameters on a pH/HCO_3^- graph will help in the diagnosis of the disorder and if the results of subsequent treatment are plotted in the same way the success of any therapy can be evaluated.

7 Acid base disturbances

Acid base disturbances can be discussed in terms of blood chemistry and there is a temptation to treat the patient rather like a test tube experiment and titrate with acid and alkali in order to correct any disturbance in blood pH. Measurement of blood pH, HCO_3^- and PCO_2 is essential in understanding any disorder but it is essential to keep in mind the clinical condition of the patient and in many instances correction of an underlying clinical disorder will restore the blood pH back to a safe level without any need to directly titrate the blood with acid or alkali infusions.

The pH/HCO_3^- diagram which was introduced in Chapter 6 has been used in the present chapter to illustrate acid base disturbances. The respiratory and renal compensation for acid base disturbances can be better understood by continual reference these diagrams and to the Henderson–Hasselbalch equation as described in Chapter 6.

Respiratory acidosis

Respiratory acidosis is an acid base disturbance related to an increase in arterial PCO_2 caused by hypoventilation. Most respiratory diseases cause hypoxia, and respiratory acidosis is less common as oxygen transport is usually disturbed rather than elimination of CO_2. Hypoxia may actually stimulate ventilation by the peripheral chemoreceptor reflex and cause respiratory alkalosis rather than respiratory acidosis. Respiratory acidosis may be caused by an overdose of drugs which depress respiration such as morphine or barbiturates; upper or lower airway obstructive disease; neuromuscular disease affecting the respiratory muscles or brain damage.

Severe acute respiratory acidosis can produce a variety of neurologic symptoms such as headache, blurred vision, restlessness and anxiety which can progress to tremors and eventually result in somnolence with CO_2 narcosis. These symptoms are not usually associated with chronic respiratory acidosis as renal compensation tends to restore blood pH back towards normal and the patient adapts to the elevated blood PCO_2.

Peripheral oedema is often associated with chronic respiratory acidosis and this may be due to the renal compensatory increase in bicarbonate reabsorption.

Mechanism of respiratory acidosis

An increase in arterial PCO_2 due to hypoventilation causes acidaemia with an increase in plasma $[H^+]$ and decrease in pH. CO_2 hydrates in the erythrocyte, in the presence of carbonic anhydrase, to form carbonic acid as follows:

$$CO_2 + H_2O \rightleftharpoons H_2CO_3 \rightleftharpoons H^+ + HCO_3^-$$

In the acute phase the H^+ formed by the above reaction is buffered almost exclusively on haemoglobin in the erythrocyte, although with chronic acidaemia, other intracellular buffers, particularly in bone become important.

An increase in arterial PCO_2 accompanied by a decrease in pH is diagnostic of respiratory acidosis. The decrease in pH is accompanied by a slight rise in plasma $[HCO_3^-]$ as HCO_3^- is the anion of carbonic acid. Carbonic acid cannot be buffered with HCO_3^- as for each H^+ formed on dissociation of carbonic acid a HCO_3^- is also generated.

The pH/HCO_3 graph illustrated in Fig. 7.1 shows the development of respiratory acidosis. An acute rise in arterial PCO_2 without any renal compensation, is illustrated by the line A–G. At point G the PCO_2 has risen to 50 mmHg with a fall in pH and an increase in $[HCO_3^-]$.

Renal compensation for respiratory acidosis

The increase in arterial PCO_2 stimulates renal compensation with a subsequent increase in H^+ secretion and HCO_3^- reabsorption as illustrated in Fig. 7.2. CO_2 has a direct effect on the renal tubule and the increased HCO_3^- reabsorption is directly related to the increase in arterial PCO_2.

Renal compensation for respiratory acidosis starts after 1–2 hours and is maximal after 2–3 days. Point H in Fig. 7.1 represents a compensated chronic respiratory acidosis. Elevation of plasma $[HCO_3^-]$ restores the ratio of PCO_2 to HCO_3^- and from the Henderson–Hasselbalch equation this will tend to restore blood pH back towards normal.

$$pH = pK + \log \frac{[HCO_3^-]}{PCO_2 \times 0.03}$$

The increased PCO_2 in respiratory acidosis is compensated by an increase in plasma $[HCO_3^-]$. The line A–H represents the situation in

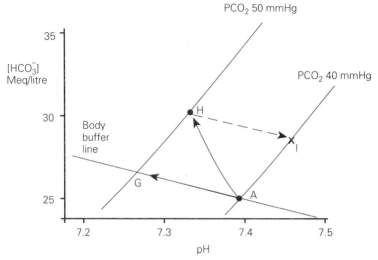

Fig. 7.1 pH/HCO$_3^-$ graph to illustrate renal compensation for respiratory acidosis. Hypoventilation with accumulation of CO$_2$ and a rise in arterial PCO$_2$ from 40–50 mm Hg is illustrated by the line A–G. A, is the normal point and G represents an acute uncompensated respiratory acidosis. Renal compensation with slow development of chronic respiratory acidosis is represented by the line A–H, as arterial PCO$_2$ increases so the kidney is stimulated to increase HCO$_3^-$ reabsorption and H$^+$ excretion. Point H represents a compensated respiratory acidosis. Point H therefore has components of respiratory acidosis and metabolic alkalosis. After renal compensation for respiratory acidosis a rapid increase in ventilation would cause a sudden change of the PCO$_2$ from PCO$_2$ 50 mm Hg at the compensated condition represented by H to PCO$_2$ 40 mm Hg represented by point I. Rapid correction of the compensated respiratory acidosis could therefore result in metabolic alkalosis as represented by point I.

which PCO$_2$ slowly increases and is accompanied by renal compensation to achieve the final compensated condition at point H.

In a condition of chronic respiratory acidosis with renal compensation the blood pH may be close to normal and a sudden reduction in arterial PCO$_2$ may be dangerous. Such a rapid reduction in PCO$_2$ is illustrated in Fig. 7.1 by the dashed line H–I where the compensated condition of respiratory acidosis at point H is changed to a condition of metabolic alkalosis at point I with an increased pH, elevated [HCO$_3^-$] and normal PCO$_2$ of 40 mm Hg. The above example demonstrates that the normal renal compensation for respiratory acidosis is equivalent to a metabolic alkalosis with elevation of plasma [HCO$_3^-$]. As long as the arterial PCO$_2$ is elevated the development of a metabolic alkalosis is an appropriate renal compensatory response as it returns the blood pH back towards pH 7.4.

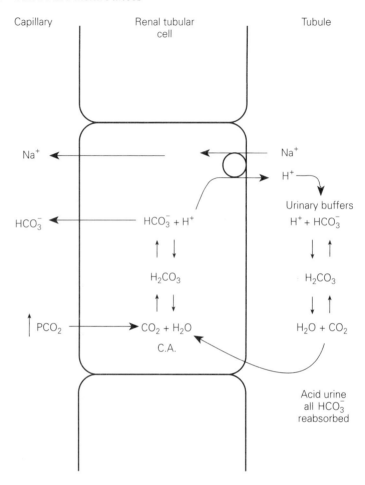

Fig. 7.2 Renal compensation for respiratory acidosis. With respiratory acidosis an increase in arterial PCO_2 stimulates H^+ secretion and HCO_3^- reabsorption in the renal tubule. CO_2 moves from the renal capillary into the renal tubular cell where it is hydrated to carbonic acid. This reaction is accelerated by the presence of carbonic anhydrase (C.A.) in the renal tubular cell. HCO_3^- reabsorption and the excretion of acid urine lead to an elevation of plasma $[HCO_3^-]$ and this renal compensation tends to return the blood pH back towards normal.

Diagnosis of respiratory acidosis

By definition any acid-base disturbance with an arterial PCO_2 greater than 40 mm Hg has a component of respiratory acidosis as shown in Fig. 6.11. An elevated arterial PCO_2 is usually accompanied by a low pH but if there has been sufficent time for renal compensation the blood pH may be close to normal. Hypoxia usually accompanies an elevated PCO_2 unless the patient is receiving oxygen, as respiratory acidosis is caused by hypoventilation. The symptoms of respiratory acidosis are non-specific, such as drowsiness, and diagnosis is dependent on the measurement of arterial blood PCO_2.

Treatment of respiratory acidosis

Treatment of respiratory acidosis involves correction of the underlying respiratory disorder. The primary aim of treatment is to restore normal ventilation. In acute respiratory acidosis supplementary oxygen and mechanical ventilation may be required to correct associated hypoxia. In chronic respiratory acidosis renal compensation is usually very effective and treatment is aimed at maintaining adequate oxygenation and improving alveolar ventilation. In treating chronic respiratory acidosis care should be taken not to cause too rapid a reduction in arterial PCO_2 by increasing ventilation as this can result in a dangerous brain alkalosis as CO_2 is readily lost from the cerebrospinal fluid but $[HCO_3^-]$ equilibrates much more slowly from the cerebrospinal fluid to the plasma.

Respiratory alkalosis

Respiratory alkalosis is caused by a decrease in arterial PCO_2 due to hyperventilation. Hyperventilation may be related to: anxiety or hysteria, hypoxia with cardiopulmonary disease or high altitude residence, elevated levels of progesterone associated with pregnancy and the luteal phase of menstrual cycle, salicylate poisoning, mechanical ventilation on a respirator, septic shock, and severe anaemia.

Symptoms of respiratory alkalosis are related to increased irritability of the central and peripheral nervous system due to alkalaemia influencing the availability of ionised Ca^{++} in extracellular fluid and cell membranes. Parasthesias, cramps, dizziness and carpopedal spasm are common symptoms. These neurologic symptoms are not usually apparent in chronic respiratory alkalosis as renal compensation tends to restore blood pH back towards normal.

Mechanism of respiratory alkalosis

A decrease in arterial PCO_2 due to hyperventilation causes alkalaemia with a decrease in plasma $[H^+]$ and increase in pH. The decrease in plasma

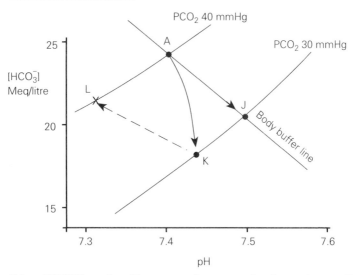

Fig. 7.3 pH/HCO3 graph to illustrate renal compensation for respiratory alkalosis. Hyperventilation with loss of CO_2 and a fall in arterial PCO_2 from 40–30 mm Hg is illustrated by the line A–J. A, is the normal point and J represents an acute uncompensated respiratory alkalosis. Renal compensation with slow development of chronic respiratory alkalosis is represented by the line A–K, as arterial PCO_2 decreases so the kidney decreases HCO_3^- reabsorption and H^+ excretion. Point K represents a compensated respiratory alkalosis. Point K therefore has components of respiratory alkalosis and metabolic acidosis. Sudden return of the PCO_2 back to 40 mm Hg from the chronic compensated condition represented by point K would result in a metabolic acidosis as shown by point L and dashed line K–L.

$[H^+]$ causes H^+ to move out of the cellular compartment and combine with HCO_3^- and reduce the plasma $[HCO_3^-]$.

The pH/HCO_3 graph illustrated in Fig. 7.3 shows the development of respiratory alkalosis. An acute decrease in arterial PCO_2 without any renal compensation is illustrated by the line A–J. At point J the PCO_2 has fallen to 30 mm Hg with a rise in pH and a decrease in $[HCO_3^-]$.

Renal compensation for respiratory alkalosis

Renal compensation for respiratory alkalosis is the mirror image of that for respiratory acidosis. Since the excretion of H^+ and reabsorption of HCO_3^- is directly related to arterial PCO_2 as shown in Fig. 7.2 a fall in PCO_2 with respiratory alkalosis causes decreased HCO_3^- reabsorption and H^+ secretion. Since H^+ secretion by the renal tubule is important for HCO_3^- reabsorption, a fall in H^+ secretion means that not all HCO_3^- is reabsorbed from the renal tubule and HCO_3^- is lost in the urine. Renal compensation for respiratory alkalosis starts after 1–2 hours and is maximal after 2–3 days. Point K in Fig. 7.3 represents a compensated chronic respiratory alkalosis. The decrease in plasma HCO_3^- has restored the ratio of PCO_2 to $[HCO_3^-]$ and from the Henderson–Hasselbalch equation this will tend to restore the pH back towards normal.

As discussed for respiratory acidosis a sudden acute change in arterial PCO_2 from the chronic compensated condition can result in a further acid base disturbance. Renal compensation for respiratory alkalosis is equivalent to development of a metabolic acidosis with a decrease in plasma $[HCO_3^-]$. A sudden return in arterial PCO_2 back towards normal from the chronic compensated condition is illustrated in Fig. 7.3 by the dashed line K–L. Point L represents a metabolic acidosis with a decreased pH, decreased $[HCO_3^-]$ and normal PCO_2 at 40 mm Hg. As long as the arterial PCO_2 is decreased below normal the development of a metabolic acidosis is an appropriate renal compensatory response as it returns the blood pH back towards pH 7.4.

Diagnosis of respiratory alkalosis

By definition any acid base disturbance with an arterial PCO_2 below 40 mm Hg has a component of respiratory alkalosis as shown in Fig. 6.11. In an acute respiratory alkalosis measurement of blood gases will reveal an alkaline pH and low PCO_2 but in chronic respiratory alkalosis the blood pH may be close to normal due to renal compensation. Chronic respiratory alkalosis with low plasma $[HCO_3^-]$ and hyperchloremia can resemble hyperchloremic metabolic acidosis except that the blood pH will be alkaline or close to normal.

Treatment of respiratory alkalosis

In general the alkalaemia associated with respiratory alkalosis is not usually life threatening and treatment is aimed at the diagnosis and correction of the underlying respiratory disorder. In acute respiratory alkalosis associated with anxiety or hysteria rebreathing into a paper bag will increase arterial PCO_2 and relieve symptoms. Hysterical hyperventilation may be treated with sedatives.

Metabolic acidosis

Metabolic acidosis is caused by accumulation of non-carbonic acid in the blood or loss of HCO_3^- and is associated with a low blood pH and low plasma $[HCO_3^-]$. Acidaemia associated with metabolic acidosis can result in potentially lethal cardiac arhythmias, lethargy and coma, and in a chronic condition cause skeletal changes due to loss of Ca^{++} and phosphate from bone. The increased blood $[H^+]$, causes compensatory hyperventilation and a fall in arterial PCO_2.

Mechanism of metabolic acidosis

Metabolic acidosis may be caused by

1. excess H^+ production – diabetes mellitus, cardiovascular shock;
2. decreased renal ability to excrete H^+ – renal failure;
3. increased loss of HCO_3^- from gut or renal tubule – diarrhoea, ureterosigmoidostomy, renal tubular acidosis.

The accumulation of non-carbonic acids in the blood such as sulphuric acid and lactic acid causes acidaemia and the blood pH is defended by four mechanisms:

1. extracellular buffering of H^+ on HCO_3^-;
2. intracellular buffering of H^+ on haemoglobin and phospates;
3. respiratory compensation with loss of CO_2;
4. renal compensation with loss of noncarbonic acid and regeneration of HCO_3^-.

These four mechanisms for the defence of blood pH in metabolic acidosis are illustrated in Fig. 7.4.

Buffering of non-carbonic acid in metabolic acidosis

The first line of defence against acidaemia on accumulation of non-carbonic acid in the blood is extracellular buffering of H^+ with HCO_3^-, and plasma $[HCO_3^-]$ may fall to as low as 10 meq/litre. Extracellular buffering will occur immediately the acid is released from the tissues and this will be followed by respiratory compensation as soon as the accumulation of H^+ in the blood is sufficent to lower blood pH below 7.4.

Over a period of hours to days there will be a movement of H^+ into the intracellular compartment and buffering on intracellular buffers such as haemoglobin, cell proteins, and phosphates. Eventually, up to 60% of the acid load may be buffered intracellularly. This intracellular shift of H^+ displaces cell cations such as K^+ and this can lead to hyperkalaemia and eventual K^+ depletion from the intracellular compartment.

Respiratory compensation in metabolic acidosis

Stimulation of peripheral arterial chemoreceptors by the increase in blood $[H^+]$ causes an increase in ventilation and a fall in arterial PCO_2. The decrease in arterial PCO_2 will tend to restore the ratio between $[HCO_3^-]$ and PCO_2 and from the Henderson–Hasselbalch equation this will return blood pH back towards normal.

$$pH = pH + \log \frac{[HCO_3^-]}{PCO_2 \times 0.03}$$

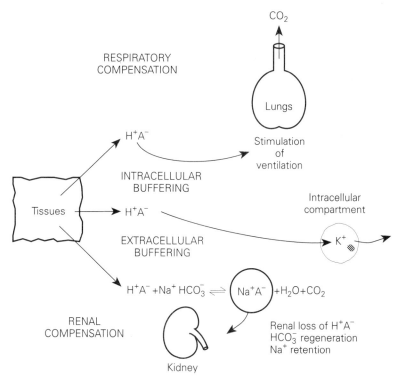

Fig. 7.4 Diagram to illustrate the factors involved in the defence of blood pH in metabolic acidosis.
An increase in the production of acid metabolites ($H^+ A^-$) by the tissues can result in metabolic acidosis. The increase in plasma [H^+] is resisted by four mechanisms; respiratory compensation, intracellular buffering, extracellular buffering, and renal compensation. The intracellular buffering of H^+ displaces K^+ from cells and this can lead to hyperkalaemia and K^+ depletion.

With severe acidaemia the stimulation of ventilation can lower arterial PCO_2 to as low as 10 mm Hg but obviously such a level of ventilation becomes exhausting after a period of hours and cannot be sustained long term.

Renal compensation for metabolic acidosis

The intracellular shift of H^+ due to acidaemia causes H^+ secretion from the kidney as accumulation of H^+ in the renal tubular cells facilitates H^+ secretion. Excretion of non-carbonic acid by the renal tubule is illustrated in Fig. 6.4 and has been discussed previously. The renal tubule secretes H^+ which accompany the anion of the acid A^- in the urine. The HCO_3^- consumed during extracellular buffering is regenerated by the renal tubule and the Na^+ ion which accompanied the acid anion A^- on filtration into the renal tubule is reabsorbed to maintain Na^+ balance. An acid urine is formed by the kidney and the renal compensatory response develops to maximum acid secretion over a period of two to three days. The limiting pH of urine is pH 4.5 and therefore only a very small fixed amount of free H^+ can be excreted each day. If daily urine volume is 1.5 litre then only 0.05 meq. of free H^+ could be excreted each day because of the limitation in pH. However, the presence of urinary buffers such as NH_3 and HCO_3^- means that the buffering capacity of the urine is capable of handling up to 500 meq of H^+ each day without exceeding the limiting pH of the renal tubule. NH_3 is produced from the metabolism of amino acids in the renal tubular cells and acidaemia enhances the production of NH_3. Stimulation of NH_3 production by acidaemia takes four to five days to reach its maximum and at this stage NH_4^+ excretion in urine can increase to more than 250 meq/day.

Metabolic acidosis and the pH/HCO_3 graph

The pH/HCO_3 graph illustrated in Fig. 7.5 shows the development of

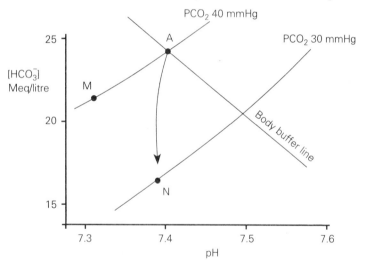

Fig. 7.5   pH/HCO_3 graph to illustrate respiratory compensation for metabolic acidosis.

Non carbonic acid (H^+A^-) formed in the tissues is buffered on HCO_3^- in extracellular fluid. Buffering of H^+ on HCO_3^- without any respiratory compensation for the acidemia is illustrated by the line A–M. Point A represents the normal condition and M is a theoretical point illustrating an uncompensated metabolic acidosis. The line A–N illustrates the actual course of metabolic acidosis with accompanying respiratory compensation. Hyperventilation lowers the PCO_2 to 30 mm Hg and the loss of carbonic acid tends to restore the blood pH back towards normal.

metabolic acidosis and subsequent respiratory compensation. Accumulation of non-carbonic acid in blood consumes HCO_3^- in extracellular fluid as H^+ are buffered on HCO_3^-. Point A represents the normal condition and the development of metabolic acidosis without renal and respiratory compensation is represented by the line A–M. Acidaemia stimulates respiration and the hyperventilation lowers arterial PCO_2. The course of the combined extracellular buffering and respiratory compensation is illustrated by the line A–N in Fig. 7.5. The blood pH is maintained near to pH 7.4 but at the expense of a great decrease in plasma $[HCO_3^-]$ and sustained hyperventilation. Renal compensation over two to three days will tend to restore plasma $[HCO_3^-]$ and excrete excess H^+, and depending on the rate of non-carbonic acid production an equilibrium will be reached between H^+ production and loss.

Standard bicarbonate

In Fig. 7.5 the respiratory compensated condition of metabolic acidosis is represented by point N. This represents a mixed metabolic acidosis/respiratory alkalosis since the respiratory compensation involves hyperventilation and a reduction in arterial PCO_2. If a blood sample is drawn from the patient in order to determine acid base status it is relatively easy to determine the involvement of any metabolic disorder by measuring *standard* HCO_3^-. The blood sample is equilibrated at PCO_2 40 mm Hg and $[HCO_3^-]$ is measured as standard $[HCO_3^-]$. If the standard $[HCO_3^-]$ is close to the normal value of 24 meq/litre then this indicates that there is no metabolic component to the acid base disturbance and that the condition is a pure respiratory disorder. If the standard $[HCO_3^-]$ differs greatly from normal then this indicates the severity of any metabolic disorder and gives a measure of base excess or base deficit. Point M in Fig. 7.5 represents a standard $[HCO_3^-]$ measurement as it lies on the PCO_2 40 mm Hg isobar. Even at PCO_2 40 mm Hg the $[HCO_3^-]$ at point M is well below normal and this is diagnostic of metabolic acidosis.

Clinical causes of metabolic acidosis

Lactic acidosis

Lactic acid is a normal product of cell metabolism and daily production is in the order of 1.4 meq/day most of which is metabolised in the liver and kidneys. Normal plasma lactate concentration is only around 0.5–1 meq/litre. Lactic acid is normally metabolised to CO_2 and H_2O or back to glucose and both of these reactions result in the regeneration of the HCO_3^- which was initially lost in buffering the lactic acid. There is normally a balance:

lactic acid production = lactic acid utilisation

Lactic acidosis is usually defined as a plasma lactate level exceeding 5 meq/litre associated with acidaemia.

The most common cause of lactic acidosis is cardiovascular shock. Lactic acid production is increased by tissue hypoxia and a shift to more anaerobic metabolism. A reduction in the perfusion of the liver caused by hypotension decreases lactic acid utilisation. Thus both sides of the equation are affected and lactic acid accumulates in the blood. A mild lactic acidosis may be associated with severe exercise where oxygen delivery to skeletal muscle cannot keep up with metabolic needs. Similarly, in grand mal epileptic seizure lactic acid production exceeds utilisation and plasma lactate levels may reach as high as 15 meq/litre.

Ketoacidosis

Diabetes mellitus is the most common cause of ketoacidosis. Insulin lack and glucagon excess cause an increase in free fatty acid delivery to the liver and altered liver metabolism, so that the fatty acids are metabolised to ketoacids rather than triglycerides. Acetoacetic acid and ß hydroxybutyric acid accumulate in the blood and cause acidaemia. Hyperglycemia usually accompanies ketoacidosis and the clinical picture may be further confused with hypovolaemia and a tendency towards cardiovascular shock.

Renal failure

Renal failure is associated with a fall in glomerular filtration rate due to a reduction in the number of functioning nephrons. This results in a metabolic acidosis due to an inability to excrete all of the daily non-carbonic acid production. An additional factor may be increased HCO_3^- loss due to reduced ability of the renal tubule to reabsorb HCO_3^-. Non-carbonic acids such as sulphuric acid accumulate in the blood and are buffered by both extracellular HCO_3^- and intracellular buffers such as bone.

Gastrointestinal loss of bicarbonate

Intestinal secretions below the stomach, including pancreatic and biliary secretions are relatively alkaline and contain high concentrations of HCO_3^-. Normally there is a balance:

$$H^+ + HCO_3^- \text{ secretions into gut} = H^+ + HCO_3^- \text{ reabsorbed from gut}$$

Loss of HCO_3^- rich secretions from the gut due to diarrhoea or the surgical drainage of pancreatic, biliary or intestinal secretions can lead to metabolic acidosis. Occasionally vomiting with intestinal obstruction can also lead to metabolic acidosis as the HCO_3^- lost in the vomit exceeds the H^+ secreted by the stomach.

Ureterosigmoidostomy, an operation which involves implantation of the ureters into the colon was previously used to drain urine after surgical removal of the bladder. Metabolic acidosis was a common postoperative complication with ureterosigmoidostomy. The colon absorbed Cl^- from the urine in exchange for HCO_3^- and this caused hyperchloremic acidosis as the HCO_3^- was lost from the colon in the faeces. Modern surgical procedures drain urine through the abdominal wall and only a small pouch of gut is used to form a reservoir for urine. With the new procedures the urine is not exposed to the large surface area of the colon and metabolic acidosis does not usually occur.

Renal tubular acidosis

Decreased ability of the kidney to excrete H^+ or reabsorb HCO_3^- may cause metabolic acidosis. There are various syndromes, particularly in infants, due to hereditary or auto-immune disease which result in metabolic acidosis due to some functional disorder in the renal tubule. Metabolic acidosis may also result from an aldosterone deficiency or failure of the renal tubule to respond to aldosterone. Since aldosterone normally stimulates H^+ and K^+ secretion, hypoaldosteronism leads to metabolic acidosis and hyperkalaemia.

Poisoning

Ingestion of acetylsalicylic acid (aspirin), ethylene glycol (an ingredient of antifreeze), methanol, and paraldehyde, cause the formation of non-carbonic acid as the substances are metabolised. Poisoning with these substances leads to metabolic acidosis.

Anion gap in metabolic acidosis

The anion gap refers to the difference between the plasma concentration of the major cation $[Na^+]$ and the combined plasma concentrations of the major anions $[Cl^-] + [HCO_3^-]$

$$[Na^+] - ([Cl^-] + [HCO_3^-]) = \text{anion gap}$$
$$140 \text{ meq/litre} - (105 \text{ meq/litre} + 24 \text{ meq/litre})$$
$$140 - 129 = 11 \text{ meq/litre}$$

The normal anion gap is around 9–14 meq/litre. Obviously this is a theoretical value as the concentrations of cations and anions in plasma must balance if electroneutrality is to be maintained. The plasma protein anions account for the anion gap as the much smaller concentrations of other ions cancel out:

$$[K^+] + [Ca^{++}] + [Mg^{++}] = [HPO_4^=] [SO_4^=], \text{ etc.}$$

On buffering of a non-carbonic acid such as H_2SO_4, HCO_3^- is consumed and replaced by the anion of the acid $SO_4^=$. If one then measures plasma $[Na^+]$, $[Cl^-]$ and $[HCO_3^-]$ and calculates the anion gap it will appear to be greater than the normal value of 11 meq/litre as the increased concentration of $SO_4^=$ is not taken into consideration by the equation. Similarly the accumulation of other anions in the plasma such as hydroxybutyrate with keto acidosis and lactate with lactic acidosis can cause an increase in the anion gap. The classification of conditions causing metabolic acidosis according to the effects on the anion gap are listed in Table 7.1.

Table 7.1   Anion gap in metabolic acidosis. With a high anion gap HCO_3^- is replaced by one of the anions A^- listed above. With a normal anion gap HCO_3^- is replaced by Cl^-.

Normal anion gap	*High anion gap*	
Loss of HCO_3^- from gut	Accumulation of non-carbonic acid (A^-)	
Diarrhoea	Keto acidosis	(ß hydroxybutyrate)
Ureterosigmoidostomy	Lactic acidosis	(lactate)
	Renal failure	($SO_4^=$ $HPO_4^=$)
	Ingestions:	
	acetyl salicylic acid	(lactate)
	ethylene glycol	(glycolate)
	menthol	(formate)
	paraldehyde	(organic anions)
	rhabdomyolysis	(organic anions)

Diarrhoea and ureterosigmoidostomy cause metabolic acidosis with a decrease in plasma $[HCO_3^-]$ but plasma Cl^- is increased in exchange for HCO_3^-. In ureterosigmoidostomy it is a direct exchange of HCO_3^- for Cl^- across the colonic mucosa and with diarrhoea the kidney retains NaCl in response to hypovolaemia and aldosterone secretion. Therefore the hyperchloremic metabolic acidosis caused by ureterosigmoidostomy and the metabolic acidosis caused by diarrhoea are associated with a normal anion gap, as the fall in plasma $[HCO_3^-]$ is balanced by a rise in $[Cl^-]$.

Diagnosis of metabolic acidosis

By definition metabolic acidosis is a plasma HCO_3^- below 24 meq/litre when arterial PCO_2 is corrected to PCO_2 40 mm Hg to give a 'standard bicarbonate'. The condition of metabolic acidosis can also be defined in terms of the pH/HCO_3^- graph, as any point plotted below the body buffer line, as illustrated in Fig. 6.11. Uncomplicated metabolic acidosis will typically be found with a low plasma $[HCO_3^-]$, low pH and with the arterial PCO_2 below normal. After determination of blood gases calculation of the anion gap in metabolic acidosis can help in the differential diagnosis of the underlying acid base disturbance as described above and shown in Table 7.1.

Treatment of metabolic acidosis

An arterial blood pH below pH 7.2 is life threatening due to the danger of cardiac depression and cardiac arhythmias. The main therapeutic aim in the treatment of metabolic acidosis is to raise the blood pH above pH 7.2 whilst monitoring plasma [K^+]. Acidaemia causes K^+ to move out of the intracellular compartment in exchange for H^+ and too rapid a decrease in plasma [H^+] can cause a sudden shift of K^+ into the intracellular compartment with serious hypokalaemia.

Intravenous $NaHCO_3$ solution is the therapy most commonly used to restore blood pH, as in metabolic acidosis plasma [HCO_3^-] is below normal. The amount of $NaHCO_3$ necessary to raise the plasma [HCO_3^-] back to a safe level cannot be calculated accurately as the acidosis is not usually a stable condition. In an emergency, with a blood pH below pH 7.2, or with apparent cardiac arhythmia, it may be prudent to inject a small volume of $NaHCO_3$ solution. Injection of $NaHCO_3$ solution can be followed by slow intravenous infusion.There are various formulae to calculate the amount of $NaHCO_3$ solution required to restore blood pH above pH 7.2 but these are only rough approximations and usually the formula has a proviso stating that only half the calculated amount should be infused slowly whilst monitoring acid base status and plasma [K^+]. The various formulae calculate the required amount of $NaHCO_3$ by making several assumptions. First, one needs to know the 'HCO_3^- space' which is the volume through which the infused HCO_3^- will equilibriate. This is often quoted as a fraction of lean body weight (0.7 x lean body weight), but it varies with acid base status and hypovolaemia. Secondly, the blood pH needs only to be raised to a safe level, above pH 7.2, and one has to estimate the plasma [HCO_3^-] in the patient that will provide a safe pH. The following formula is often quoted:

$$HCO_3^- \text{ deficit} = HCO_3^- \text{ space x } HCO_3^- \text{ deficit/litre}$$

$$HCO_3^- \text{ deficit} = (0.7 \text{ x lean bodyweight}) \text{ x } (10 - \text{actual plasma } HCO_3^-)$$

The actual plasma [HCO_3^-] is subtracted from 10 as it is only necessary to raise the plasma [HCO_3^-] to a safe level of 10 meq/litre. The formula gives the clinician a starting point but it does not really offer much advantage over slowly infusing $NaHCO_3$ and carefully monitoring acid base status.

In lactic acidosis associated with cardiovascular shock the use of intravenous $NaHCO_3$ solution is controversial as buffering of lactic acid will release CO_2 as HCO_3^- is consumed, and the CO_2 released in the tissues could cause a rapid fall in intracellular pH. CO_2 readily crosses cell membranes and influences intracellular pH and can also easily enter cerebrospiral fluid and cause depression of the central nervous system. Therefore the first line of therapy in cardiovascular shock is to restore blood volume and blood pressure, and the lactic acidosis will correct itself once tissue hypoxia is controlled. Excessive $NaHCO_3$ infusion in metabolic acidosis associated with cardiovascular shock could cause a swing from metabolic acidosis to metabolic alkalosis with hypokalaemia.

In ketoacidosis associated with diabetes mellitus insulin is the therapy of choice as it will correct the acidosis by causing metabolism of the ketoacids to CO_2 and H_2O and regeneration of HCO_3^-. Therapy with $NaHCO_3$ solution is controversial as it can easily precipitate alkalaemia and hypokalaemia. Insulin causes a shift of extracellular K^+ towards the intracellular compartment and if this is accompanied by alkalaemia there will be a further shift of K^+ intracellularly which could cause dangerous hypokalaemia.

The metabolic acidosis associated with renal failure is usually well tolerated in the adult, and with respiratory compensation the blood pH stabilises above pH 7.2. Intravenous infusion of $NaHCO_3$ may precipitate tetany if hypocalcemia is already established and in acute renal failure excessive intravenous administration of fluids can cause a dangerous hypervolaemia.

In diarrhoea, correction of hypovolaemia may be the first therapeutic aim. Acidaemia is likely to be accompanied by K^+ depletion and it is essential to follow plasma $[K^+]$ concentration as acidaemia is corrected. In the hypokalaemic patient with acidaemia $NaHCO_3$ and KCl must be administered concurrently with careful monitoring of blood pH, plasma $[K^+]$ and electrocardiograph. Again as with all of the above treatments the therapeutic goal should be to raise the blood pH above pH 7.2 rather than attempt to restore blood pH back to normal. Once the blood pH is at a safe level treatment of the underlying disorder will tend to correct the blood pH further towards normal.

Metabolic alkalosis

Metabolic alkalosis is primarily related to a high plasma $[HCO_3^-]$ and high blood pH. The neurologic symptoms of alkalosis such as dizziness, carpopedal spasm and parasthesias are not as common in metabolic alkalosis as respiratory alkalosis. This may be because the anion HCO_3^- does not penetrate cell membranes and the cerebro spinal fluid as easily as CO_2. Patients with metabolic alkalosis may be asymptomatic or complain of symptoms more related to hypovolaemia and hypokalaemia such as postural hypotension, muscle weakness, polyuria and polydipsia.

Mechanism of metabolic alkalosis

The kidney has a great capacity to excrete HCO_3^- and in order for metabolic alkalosis to be sustained two requirements must be met: first, a mechanism for increasing extracellular $[HCO_3^-]$; secondly, a mechanism to prevent the kidney from excreting the excess HCO_3^-. The two mechanisms must operate together as merely preventing the kidney from excreting HCO_3^-, e.g. anuria does not result in metabolic alkalosis.

The extracellular $[HCO_3^-]$ may be increased by either H^+ loss or HCO_3^- retention.

H+ loss may be due to:
    vomiting – GIT loss of H^+;
    hyperaldosteronism – renal loss of H^+;
    diuretics – renal loss of H^+;
    hypokalaemia – intracellular shift of H^+, renal loss of H^+.

HCO3- retention may be due to:
    massive blood transfusion – citrate metabolised to HCO_3^-;
    infusion of $NaHCO_3$ – therapeutic error;
    milk alkali syndrome – chronic ingestion of milk and antacid.

The plasma $[HCO_3^-]$ can also be increased by diuretic treatment which may cause a contraction of the extracellular fluid compartment without loss of HCO_3^-. This is sometimes referred to as a 'contraction alkalosis'.

As mentioned above, merely increasing the plasma $[HCO_3^-]$ is not sufficent to induce metabolic alkalosis and there must also be an increase in the renal threshold for HCO_3^- excretion. Normally HCO_3^- is excreted in the urine once the plasma $[HCO_3^-]$ exceeds 28 meq/litre. The renal threshold for HCO_3^- excretion can be increased by several factors such as hypovolaemia, hypercalcemia, hypokalaemia and hypochloraemia. The role of these factors in sustaining metabolic alkalosis will be discussed below.

Elevation of plasma $[HCO_3^-]$ causes alkalaemia and the blood pH is defended by three mechanisms:

1.   shift of H^+ from intracellular to extracellular compartment;
2.   respiratory compensation – hypoventilation with elevation of arterial PCO_2;
3.   renal compensation – with loss of HCO_3^- and decreased H^+ secretion.

Unlike metabolic acidosis where the respiratory and renal compensatory responses significantly limit the change in blood pH, in metabolic alkalosis the compensatory responses are limited and the excess HCO_3^- is mainly buffered by movement of H^+ from the intracellular to the extracellular compartment.

Respiratory compensation in metabolic alkalosis

Respiratory compensation for alkalaemia involves hypoventilation and retention of CO_2 to form carbonic acid. The hypoventilation is caused by a decreased [H$^+$] around peripheral arterial chemoreceptors. However, the respiratory compensation is very limited, as hypoventilation results in hypoxia and this is a potent stimulus for ventilation. Because of the braking effect of hypoxia on the hypoventilatory response the arterial PCO_2 rarely exceeds PCO_2 55 mmHg and in many cases respiratory compensation is not apparent.

Renal compensation for metabolic alkalosis

The kidney has a great capacity to excrete HCO_3^- and with normal renal function metabolic alkalosis cannot be sustained for long as renal compensation would lead to excretion of excess HCO_3^- and formation of an alkaline urine. Renal compensation is brought about by a decrease in plasma [H$^+$] causing a decrease in renal H$^+$ secretion. Since H$^+$ secretion is necessary for HCO_3^- reabsorption, the decrease in renal H$^+$ secretion causes a decrease in HCO_3^- reabsorption and loss of HCO_3^- in urine. With normal renal function only a mild and short-lived metabolic alkalosis would develop. As will be discussed below treatment of metabolic alkalosis is often aimed at restoring normal renal function and subsequent excretion of HCO_3^-.

pH/ HCO_3^- diagram and metabolic alkalosis

The pH/ HCO_3^- diagram in Fig. 7.6 illustrates the development of metabolic alkalosis caused for example by prolonged vomiting. The normal condition is represented by point A and the development of metabolic alkalosis is illustrated by the arrow to point O. Point O represents a condition of metabolic alkalosis with an increase in plasma [HCO_3^-] concentration and an increase in pH, without any renal or respiratory compensation. In order for this increase in plasma [HCO_3^-] to be sustained there must be some limitation on the ability of the kidney to excrete HCO_3^-. Therefore renal compensation cannot occur without treatment of the associated hypovolaemia and electrolyte disorders as described below. Correction of the renal problem would cause HCO_3^- excretion and formation of an alkali urine and a return towards the normal pH 7.4. Respiratory compensation for metabolic alkalosis involves a depression of respiration and hypoventilation. The depression of respiration is due to a decrease in [H$^+$] around the peripheral arterial chemoreceptors. The subsequent respiratory hypoventilation causes retention of CO_2 which tends to return the blood pH back towards normal. Respiratory compensation for metabolic alkalosis is shown in Fig. 7.6 by the line A–P which represents the development of metabolic alkalosis and subsequent respiratory compensation. Point P represents the compensated condition with an elevated PCO_2 of 50 mm Hg. Note that the respiratory compensation actually causes a further rise in plasma HCO_3^- concentration as HCO_3^- is the anion of carbonic acid. The

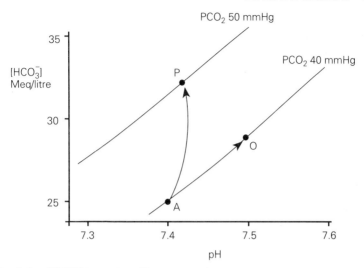

Fig. 7.6 pH/HCO3 graph to illustrate respiratory compensation for metabolic alkalosis.
The normal condition is represented by point A and metabolic alkalosis without repiratory compensation by point O. The line A–P represents the normal path with the development of metabolic alkalosis and simultaneous respiratory compensation. Hypoventilation causes an increase in arterial PCO_2 and subsequent increase in carbonic acid. The increase in PCO_2 maintains the ratio between CO_2 and HCO_3^- and returns the pH back towards normal despite an increase in plasma HCO_3^-.

respiratory compensation causes blood pH to move towards normal because the ratio between CO_2 and HCO_3^- is corrected by an increase in CO_2. In most conditions of metabolic alkalosis the respiratory compensation is very limited and the arterial PCO_2 is close to normal.

Clinical causes of metabolic alkalosis

Metabolic alkalosis caused by vomiting

Vomiting is the most common cause of metabolic alkalosis. Secretion of HCl in the stomach is accompanied by secretion of HCO_3^- into the blood, the alkaline tide. Normally the gastric acid would be neutralised in the duodenum by pancreatic and biliary secretions rich in HCO_3^- but if the acid is lost from the stomach by vomiting or nasogastric suction then there is no stimulus for pancreatic and biliary secretions. The result is that HCO_3^- accumulates in the blood and causes metabolic alkalosis. The excess plasma HCO_3^- is not readily excreted in the urine because of changed renal function due to three conditions resulting from vomiting: hypovolaemia, hypokalaemia and hypochloraemia.

Hypovolaemia is caused by fluid loss due to vomiting. The hypovolaemia leads to aldosterone secretion with renal retention of Na⁺, and loss of H⁺ and K⁺ in exchange for Na⁺.

Hypokalaemia is caused by increased renal loss of K⁺ due to raised levels of aldosterone, intracellular alkalosis, decreased K⁺ intake and loss of K⁺ secretions in vomit. Intracellular alkalosis of renal tubular cells is the major mechanism causing hypokalaemia as in the presence of aldosterone K⁺ is lost in exchange for Na⁺ if H⁺ is not readily available for exchange. With prolonged vomiting a reduction in K⁺ intake and an increase in K⁺ loss may also contribute to hypokalaemia.

Hypochloremia is caused by loss of Cl⁻ in the HCl in vomit together with decreased Cl⁻ intake.

The development of metabolic alkalosis due to vomiting is illustrated in Fig. 7.7. Vomiting causes hypovolaemia and the subsequent renal response of Na⁺ retention limits excretion of excess HCO_3^-.

The renal response is critical in the development of metabolic alkalosis

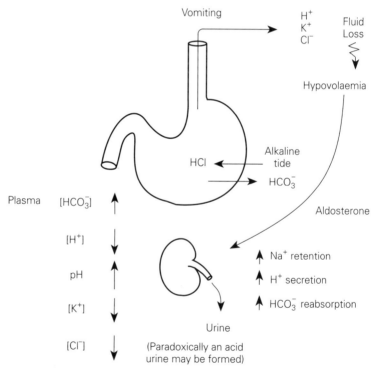

Fig. 7.7   Diagram to illustrate the factors involved in the development of metabolic alkalosis caused by vomiting. Vomiting causes metabolic alkalosis due to loss of acid from the stomach and accumulation of HCO_3^- in the blood. The associated hypovolaemia, hypokalaemia and hypochloraemia alter renal function so that the excess plasma HCO_3^- is not readily excreted in the urine.

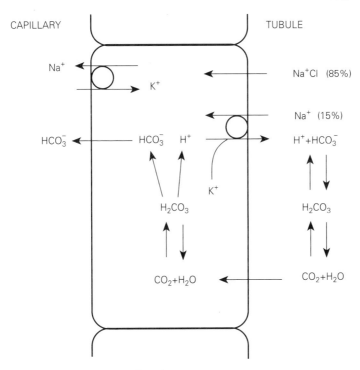

Fig. 7.8 Renal handling of Na$^+$. Na$^+$ is reabsorbed from the renal tubule together with an accompanying anion. Normally 85% of Na$^+$ is reabsorbed with Cl$^-$ and 15% with HCO$_3^-$. Reabsorption of Na$^+$ with HCO$_3^-$ is accomplished by H$^+$ secretion and to a lesser extent K$^+$ secretion. The ability of the renal tubule to excrete excess HCO$_3^-$ in metabolic alkalosis may be restricted by three factors which favour H$^+$ secretion and reabsorption of HCO$_3^-$; hypokalaemia, hypovolaemia, and hypochloraemia. The influence of these three factors on renal handling of HCO$_3^-$ is discussed in the text.

as instead of excreting HCO$_3^-$ there is increased HCO$_3^-$ reabsorption by the kidney in response to increased Na$^+$ retention, increased H$^+$ secretion, hypokalaemia and hypochloraemia. In order to understand this paradoxical renal response it is necessary to examine renal function in some more detail as illustrated in Fig. 7.8. Na$^+$ is reabsorbed from the renal tubule together with an accompanying anion. Normally 85% of reabsorbed Na$^+$ is accompanied with Cl$^-$ and 15% with HCO$_3^-$. Reabsorption of Na$^+$ with HCO$_3^-$ is accompanied by H$^+$ secretion. In metabolic alkalosis accompanied by hypovalaemia the increased secretion of aldosterone stimulates Na$^+$ reabsorption. Because of the increased plasma [HCO$_3^-$] and decreased [Cl$^-$] a much greater fraction of the filtered Na$^+$ is accompanied by HCO$_3^-$. Reabsorption of Na$^+$ with HCO$_3^-$ involves H$^+$ secretion and paradoxically the alkalaemia may be accompanied by formation of acid urine.

Acid secretion from the renal tubule is also facilitated by the concomitant hypokalaemia. Normally in the presence of aldosterone some of the filtered Na^+ which is exchanged for H^+ could be reabsorbed in exchange for K^+ but with hypokalaemia this Na^+/K^+ exchange is restricted. Thus hypokalaemia will also favour H^+ secretion by the renal tubule.

Contraction alkalosis

Contraction alkalosis is caused by a reduction in the extracellular fluid volume without concomitant loss of HCO_3^-. This condition may be caused by the use of potent diuretics such as ethacrynic acid in the treatment of congestive heart failure. The extracellular fluid compartment contracts as water is lost and the $[HCO_3^-]$ is increased in the remaining fluid.

Milk alkali syndrome

Milk alkali syndrome refers to metabolic alkalosis caused by excessive intake of milk and alkali antacids. The syndrome is associated with hypercalcaemia and in the chronic condition there may be abnormal calcification of bone. The alkalosis is due to excessive intake of alkali and a reduced ability of the renal system to excrete HCO_3^-. Hypercalcaemia causes enhanced HCO_3^- reabsorpton by the proximal renal tubule and this sustains the metabolic alkalosis.

Diagnosis of metabolic acidosis

By definition metabolic alkalosis is a plasma $[HCO_3^-]$ above 24 meq/litre when arterial PCO_2 is corrected to PCO_2 40 mm Hg (standard HCO_3^- greater than 24 meq/litre) , as illustrated in Fig. 6.11. Any arterial blood pH greater than 7.4 can be defined as alkalaemia but alkalosis is usually associated with a blood pH greater than pH 7.44. The differential diagnosis will depend on clinical history to identify cases of vomiting, diuretic therapy, nasogastric suction and milk alkali syndrome. Hypovolaemia is a common mechanism for the maintenance of metabolic alkalosis and is often associated with a low urinary Cl^- concentration (<10 meq/litre). Urinary Cl^- is a better index of volume status than Na^+ in hypovolaemia associated with metabolic alkalosis, as urinary Na^+ may be maintained at a high level despite hypovolaemia as Na^+ is excreted in urine as a cation accompanying excess HCO_3^-.

Treatment of metabolic alkalosis

The alkalaemia associated with metabolic alkalosis is only rarely treated by the infusion of acid. The kidney can normally excrete HCO_3^- to correct alkalaemia and the aim of therapy is to restore renal function by treating associated hypovolaemia, hypokalaemia and hypochloraemia. Once renal function is restored to normal an alkali urine is formed and blood pH moves towards pH 7.4.

Hypovolaemia and hypochloremia can be treated by infusion of NaCl as isotonic or half isotonic solution. It is important that the Na^+ is accompanied by Cl^- as the anion, as Na^+ will then be reabsorbed from the renal tubule as NaCl. Administration of Na^+ with any other anion, e.g. $SO_4^=$ would restrict Na^+ reabsorption by the the renal tubule to exchange of Na^+ for H^+. This would therefore perpetuate H^+ secretion and HCO_3^- regeneration as illustrated in Figs 7.2 and 7.8.

Metabolic alkalosis caused by loss of acid due to vomiting/drainage or diuretics is termed *saline responsive* alkalosis as the alkalosis is sustained due to altered renal function caused by hypovolaemia and hypochloraemia. Saline responsive alkalosis, as the name implies, can be treated by infusion of NaCl. *Saline resistant alkalosis* is typically caused by K^+ depletion. Infusion of KCl solution corrects the alkalosis in three ways:

1. allows increased HCO_3^- excretion as K^+ is lost from renal tubule instead of H^+;
2. allows Na^+ reabsorption with Cl^- and reduces the fraction of Na^+ reabsorbed in exchange for H^+;
3. causes H^+ to move from the intracellular to the extracellular compartment.

Saline resistant alkalosis is associated with K^+ depletion rather than hypovolaemia but with vomiting the hypovolaemia may also be combined with K^+ loss and therefore KCl will be required as well as NaCl to treat the metabolic alkalosis.

Congestive heart failure and various oedematous conditions are often associated with metabolic alkalosis due to diuretic therapy and in these cases therapy with acetazolamide is preferred as this increases the renal excretion of $NaHCO_3$.

Direct titration of HCO_3^- with acid can be used to treat metabolic alkalosis and ammonium chloride and HCl have been used. Acid titration is usually reserved for acute cases of severe alkalaemia accompanied by hypervolaemia. Administration of HCl as an infusion is a problem because of the irritancy of the acid, and if the acid is administered in a very dilute solution then volume overload may occur. HCl should only be administered by a central venous line and the aim should be to return blood pH back to a safe level of less than pH 7.45. Titration of HCO_3^- may also cause dilution of plasma and subsequent hyponatraemia as there is no gain of solute on reaction of $NaHCO_3$ with HCl.

Mixed acid base disturbances

Mixed acid base disturbances are common and interpretation is helped by plotting the disorder on a pH/HCO_3^- graph. A mixed disorder could be represented by the following arterial blood gas parameters; pH = 7.3, PCO_2 = 50 mm Hg, [HCO_3^-] = 35 meq/litre. This is a relatively mild acid base disturbance as the pH is above the clinically dangerous level of pH 7.2 and it represents the situation one might see in a compensated disorder. The acid base disorder could be related to renal compensation for a primary disorder of respiratory acidosis or respiratory compensation for a primary disorder of metabolic alkalosis.

In this mild acid base disturbance only the clinical history will be able to indicate whether the underlying acid base disturbance is of respiratory or metabolic origin. If the arterial PCO_2 was much greater than PCO_2 50 mmHg then the primary disorder would be a respiratory acidosis as respiratory compensation for metabolic acidosis is limited by hypoxia and rarely exceeds PCO_2 55 mmHg.

Respiratory acidosis and respiratory alkalosis cannot coexist but metabolic acidosis and metabolic alkalosis can be found together. Here it is important to stress that the terms acidosis and alkalosis refer to the underlying disorder and that the blood pH and [HCO_3^-] may be high, low or normal depending on the predominance of one disorder or the other. In general the PCO_2 will adjust according to the [HCO_3^-] and pH but it is possible for a third component of repiratory acidosis or alkalosis to coexist with the two metabolic disorders. Diagnosis of the disorders will depend on the clinical history.

Summary

The carbonic acid–bicarbonate buffering system is central to acid base disturbances as all disturbances can be explained by some change in the ratio between carbonic acid and bicarbonate as related to the Henderson–Hasselbalch equation.

$$pH = pK + \log \frac{[HCO_3^-]}{PCO_2 \times 0.03}$$

The respiratory and renal compensatory responses correct the ratio not necessarily the absolute amounts of carbonic acid and HCO_3^-, and therefore defend the blood pH.

A summary of acid base disturbances together with renal and respiratory compensations is given in Table 7.2. In all cases the respiratory and renal compensatory responses tend to bring blood pH back towards normal by restoring the ratio of carbonic acid to HCO_3^-.

The common causes of acid-base disturbance are summarised in Table 7.3.

Table 7.2 Summary acid base disturbances. The primary acid base disturbance is indicated by the solid arrow and secondary respiratory and renal compensatory responses by the dashed arrow.

	pH	[H⁺]	PCO₂	[HCO⁻₃]	Compensation Respiratory	Renal
Respiratory acidosis	↓	↑	↑ (solid)	↑ (dashed)	None	HCO⁻₃ retention
Metabolic acidosis	↓	↑	↓ (dashed)	↓ (solid)	PCO₂ ↓	HCO⁻₃ retention
Respiratory alkalosis	↑	↓	↓ (solid)	↓ (dashed)	None	HCO⁻₃ excretion
Metabolic alkalosis	↑	↓	↑ (dashed)	↑ (solid)	PCO₂ ↑	HCO⁻₃ excretion

Table 7.3 Common causes of acid base disturbance

Respiratory alkalosis	Respiratory acidosis	Metabolic alkalosis	Metabolic acidosis
Hypoxia	Obstructive airway disease	*Acid loss*	Diabetes mellitus
Hysteria	CNS depressant overdose	Vomiting	Cardiovascular shock
Anxiety	Brain damage	Gastric aspiration	Renal failure
Pregnancy	Neuromuscular disease	Alkali infusion/ ingestion	Diarrhoea
Progesterone Artificial ventilation Salicylate overdose Septicaemia	Artificial ventilation	*Potassium loss* Vomiting Diuretics Hyperaldosteronism	Ingestion – salicylate, methanol, ethylene glycol, etc.

8 Potassium homeostasis; hypokalaemia and hyperkalaemia

Nearly all of the body K^+ is found within the intracellular compartment and K^+ is actively transported into cells in exchange for Na^+ as shown in Fig. 8.1. Because most of the body store of K^+ is found within the intracellular compartment the plasma $[K^+]$ is often unrelated to the level of body stores of K^+.

The intracellular $[K^+]$ is much greater than extracellular $[K^+]$ and because the cell membrane is relatively permeable to K^+, K^+ moves down a concentration gradient out of the cell. Continuous diffusion of K^+ out of the cell creates the resting cell membrane potential of –70 to –90 mv.

In vitro an increase of extracellular $[K^+]$ causes depolarisation of the cell membrane potential from -70 mv towards 0. Initially this depolarisation can excite the cell as the cell membrane approaches threshold but when the cell membrane potential is maintained in a depolarised state

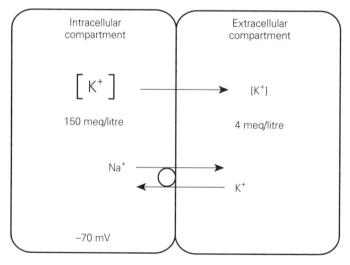

Fig. 8.1 Intracellular K^+. The intracellular $[K^+]$ is maintained by active transport of K^+ in exchange for Na^+. The resting cell membrane is relatively permeable to K^+ but not to Na^+. K^+ moves down a concentration gradient out of the cell and establishes the resting cell membrane at –70 to –90 mV.

decreased excitability of the cell occurs. *In vitro* a decrease of extracellular [K⁺] causes an increase in the resting membrane potential well above threshold value and this stabilises the membrane potential and decreases cell excitability.

In vivo changes in plasma [K⁺] with hypokalaemia and hyperkalaemia cause changes in the activity of excitable tissues such as nerve and cardiac muscle with symptoms such as muscle weakness and cardiac arhythmias.

Body K⁺ stores are maintained relatively constant at 3–4 equivalents of K⁺ and this large intracellular store of K⁺ is in equilibrium with the small amount of K⁺ in extracellular fluid. The plasma [K⁺] is held constant at around 4 meq/litre by exchange with the intracellular compartment and by renal regulation. Factors influencing plasma [K⁺] are illustrated in Fig. 8.2. There is a balance between K⁺ and H⁺ as intracellular cations and an increase in the extracellular [H⁺] with acidaemia causes H⁺ to enter cells and displace K⁺. Alkalaemia has the reverse effect and causes K⁺ to move from the extracellular to the intracellular compartment. Insulin, glucose and adrenaline cause K⁺ movement into the intracellular compartment and administration of insulin can cause hypokalaemia.

Normally there is more than adequate K⁺ intake as foods such as meat, vegetables, etc., are cellular and contain K⁺. There is usually no problem with excessive K⁺ intake if renal function is normal as the kidneys readily

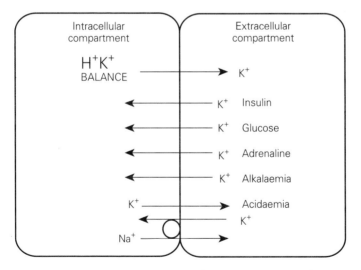

Fig. 8.2 Factors influencing extracellular [K⁺]. The extracellular [K⁺] is kept low by active transport of K⁺ into the intracellular compartment. There is a balance between [K⁺] and [H⁺] in the cell and an increase in extracellular [H⁺] with acidaemia causes H⁺ to enter the cells and displace K⁺. Alkalaemia has the opposite effect and causes K⁺ to move from the extracellular to the intracellular compartment. Insulin , glucose and adrenaline cause K⁺ movent into the intracellular compartment and the administration of insulin can cause hypokalaemia.

excrete excess K^+. The balance between K^+ intake and loss is regulated by K^+ secretion in the renal collecting tubules. Renal K^+ secretion is influenced by two factors:

1. aldosterone secretion from the adrenal cortex;
2. plasma $[K^+]$ and K^+ exchange with the intracellular compartment.

An increase in plasma $[K^+]$ directly stimulates release of aldosterone from the adrenal cortex. Aldosterone stimulates renal secretion of K^+ by increasing the activity of the peritubular Na^+/K^+ pump and by increasing the permeability of the luminal membrane to K^+. Similarly an increase in plasma $[K^+]$ causes an intracellular shift of K^+ and promotes K^+ secretion from the renal tubular cell as illustrated in Fig. 8.3. The K^+ secretion is essentially passive and depends on the concentration gradient from the renal tubular cell to the tubular fluid. Increased renal tubular flow as with a diuresis promotes K^+ secretion by 'wash out' of K^+.

K^+ and H^+ ions can also be exchanged for Na^+ at the luminal membrane,

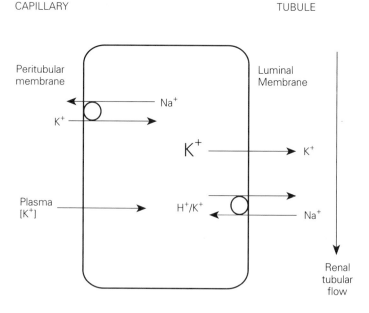

Fig. 8.3   Factors influencing secretion of K^+ from collecting tubule. K^+ moves out of the renal tubular cell into the tubular fluid down a concentration gradient. This passive secretion of K^+ is increased by aldosterone which stimulates the peritubular Na^+/K^+ pump and increases the permeability of the luminal membrane for K^+. An increase in plasma $[K^+]$ similarly favours K^+ secretion by promoting an intra cellular shift of K^+. Increased renal tubular flow promotes K^+ secretion by 'wash out' of K^+.

with active transport causing increased Na^+ reabsorption. Normally around 15% of the filtered Na^+ is reabsorbed in exchange for H^+ or K^+ with 85% of Na^+ passively reabsorbed across the luminal membrane along with Cl^-.

The renal exchange of K^+ for Na^+ is stimulated by aldosterone which regulates plasma K^+ concentration. Aldosterone also stimulates Na^+ uptake and K^+ loss across the colonic mucosa.

Hypokalaemia

Hypokalaemia can be caused by a deficient intake of K^+ and excessive renal or gastro-intestinal loss of K^+. Since a normal diet contains more than sufficent K^+ a reduction in K^+ intake is usually related to prolonged vomiting rather than dietary deficiency.

Clinical causes of hypokalaemia

Excessive renal loss of K^+ is often associated with diuresis as the increased renal tubular flow tends to wash K^+ out of renal tubular cells. Administration of diuretics or an osmotic diuresis with glycosuria can therefore lead to hypokalaemia. Diuretics may be administered with a K^+ supplement in order to prevent hypokalaemia but the increase in K^+ intake is frequently insufficent to prevent a mild hypokalaemia. Renal tubular disease and conditions such as Conn's syndrome and Cushing's syndrome with mineralocorticoid excess can also cause hypokalaemia by stimulating renal K^+ secretion.

Excessive loss of K^+ from the gastro-intestinal tract is associated with diarrhoea and inflammatory bowel disease. The secretions of the gastro-intestinal tract contain K^+, and with diarrhoea, daily stool losses of K^+ may be greatly increased.

Mild hypokalaemia may also occur with alkalaemia as this causes a shift of H^+ out of the intracellular compartment in exchange for an inward movement of K^+ from plasma.

Vomiting can cause hypokalaemia by loss of K^+ in the vomit together with decreased potassium intake. Alkalaemia and hypovolaemia associated with vomiting exacerbate the hypokalaemia by first causing a shift of K^+ into the cellular compartment and secondly stimulating aldosterone secretion and renal reabsorption of Na^+ in exchange for K^+.

Hyperaldosteronism caused by hyperplasia of the adrenal gland causes hypokalaemia but the K^+ loss is dependent on adequate delivery of Na^+ to the distal renal tubule.

Aldosterone secretion is increased on a low salt diet and with congestive heart failure but this does not cause K^+ loss and hypokalaemia as there is an increase in renal Na^+ reabsorption and the distal delivery of Na^+ is reduced. Hypokalaemia is commonly found in patients with congestive heart failure when they are treated with a diuretic as this increases distal

Na^+ delivery in the renal tubule and allows K^+ exchange for Na^+. If these patients were only treated with a low salt diet they would not develop hypokalaemia even though aldosterone levels were increased.

Diagnosis of hypokalaemia

Symptoms of hypokalaemia may be apparent when plasma $[K^+]$ falls below 2.5–3 meq/litre and these include muscle weakness, cardiac arhythmias, electrocardiograph (ECG) changes and impaired renal concentrating function with polyuria and polydipsia. Severe hypokalaemia can lead to muscle paralysis and respiratory failure.

Hypokalaemia produces characteristic changes in the ECG as shown in Fig. 8.4 mainly due to delayed ventricular repolarisation. The ECG shows S–T segment depression associated with decreased amplitude or inversion of the T wave and increased amplitude of the U wave.

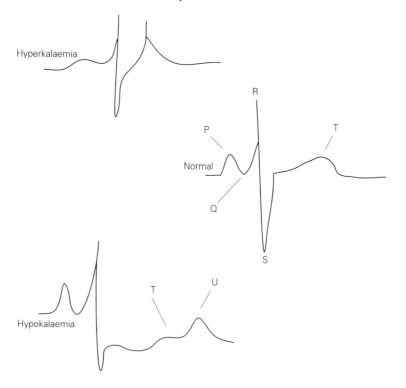

Fig, 8.4   The effects of changes in extracellular $[K^+]$ on the electrocardiograph. Hyperkalaemia causes changes in the e.c.g. with decreased amplitude of the P wave and a peaked T wave. Hypokalaemia causes delayed ventricular repolarisation with the e.c.g. showing depression of the S–T segment and increased amplitude of the U wave.

Treatment of hypokalaemia

Treatment of hypokalaemia is via oral or intravenous therapy with K^+ salts. The first step is to determine the severity of the hypokalaemia by assessing cardiac and muscle symptoms. There is a wide variety of response to hypokalaemia and the severity of cardiac and muscle symptoms is often unrelated to the magnitude of the hypokalaemia, especially if onset of hypokalaemia has been very slow.

Oral KCl can be given in the majority of patients with mild to moderate hypokalaemia and plasma $[K^+]$ ranging from 2.7–3.5 meq/litre. In patients who are unable to eat or with severe life-threatening cardiac symptoms intravenous therapy is necessary. KCl infusion can rapidly correct hypokalaemia and improve symptoms but correction of K^+ depletion may require multiple infusions as K^+ moves from the extracellular to the intracellular compartment. Concentrations of KCl greater than 40–60 meq/litre should not be used as they may cause irritation and sclerosis of the vein. This limit on the upper concentration of KCl solutions means that it is often difficult to correct a long standing K^+ deficit by intravenous therapy as large volumes of fluid are required.

K^+ solutions should be infused slowly with monitoring of muscle strength and ECG as hypokalaemia can easily be reversed to a life-threatening hyperkalaemia with rapid infusions.

Hyperkalaemia

Hyperkalaemia is only rarely associated with excessive K^+ intake if renal function is normal. Excess K^+ readily enters the cellular compartment and any increase in plasma K^+ concentration is normally resisted by renal excretion of K^+. Hyperkalaemia is caused by renal failure, inappropriate use of K^+ sparing diuretics, hypoaldosteronism and insulin deficiency associated with hyperglycemia.

Although hyperkalaemia is not normally found due to excessive dietary intake of K^+ it is sometimes caused by therapeutic error in the administration of K^+ salts intravenously for the treatment of hypokalaemia. K^+ salts should always be used with caution if there is any reason to suspect impaired renal function as in these patients K^+ loads that would normally be well tolerated may lead to dangerous elevation of plasma $[K^+]$. Chronic hyperkalaemia is always associated with impaired renal function since K^+ is readily excreted by the normal kidney. Hyperkalaemia is uncommon until over 90% of renal function is lost and GFR is less than 20%.

Diagnosis of hyperkalaemia

Hyperkalaemia can be defined as a plasma $[K^+]$ greater than the upper laboratory limit of normal and this is usually in excess of 5.5 meq/litre.

Symptoms of hyperkalaemia are basically limited to muscle weakness and abnormal cardiac conduction leading to arhythimias. Cardiac abnormalities may be apparent once the plasma [K$^+$] exceeds 6 meq/litre and muscle weakness generally is found once [K$^+$] exceeds 8 meq/litre. The ECG changes are illustrated in Fig. 8.4 and are initially a peaked T wave and with more severe hyperkalaemia a widening of the QRS complex and decreased amplitude and eventually complete loss of the P wave. Spurious elevation of plasma [K$^+$] may be caused by haemolysis of the blood sample and pseudohyperkalaemia should be ruled out before initiating treatment.

Treatment of hyperkalaemia

Treatment of hyperkalaemia depends on the severity of muscle and cardiac symptoms and the nature of the underlying disorder. A plasma [K$^+$] greater than 8 meq/litre with signs of muscle weakness associated with ECG changes requires immediate action. Hyperkalemia tends to depolarise cell membranes and this effect can be antagonised by increasing the plasma [Ca^{++}]. The administration of calcium gluconate returns membrane excitability towards normal and protects against hyperkalaemia. Calcium gluconate has a rapid onset of action but the protective effect is short lived. The plasma [K$^+$] can also be lowered by causing a shift of K$^+$ towards the intracellular compartment. In diabetics the administration of insulin causes a decrease in plasma [K$^+$] by causing K$^+$ to enter the intracellular compartment. In uncontrolled diabetes there is a danger of severe hypokalaemia with insulin treatment, as insulin may cause a rapid intracellular shift of K$^+$. In non-diabetics hyperkalaemia may be treated by administration of insulin together with glucose to cause an intracellular shift of K$^+$. The administration of NaHCO$_3$ solution causes an intracellular shift in K$^+$ by facilitating exchange of K$^+$ for intracellular H$^+$ and this is particularly effective when hyperkalaemia is associated with metabolic acidosis.

The effects of Ca^{++}, insulin and NaHCO$_3$ are short lived and K$^+$ that has been shifted intracellularly will tend to return to the extracellular compartment over several hours. Long-term treatment for persistent hyperkalaemia must involve removal of excess K$^+$ from the body by the use of diuretics and renal dialysis.

Pseudohyperkalaemia, pseudohypokalaemia

Pseudohyperkalaemia is a false elevation of plasma [K$^+$] occurring during the *in vitro* handling of a blood sample. The [K$^+$] is high in red blood cells and haemolysis caused by damage during venepuncture or later whilst handling the sample can result in pseudohyperkalaemia. Typically the serum will have a red tint due to the presence of haemoglobin released from the damaged red cells. K$^+$ can also be released from platelets and leukocytes especially during clotting and a false elevation of plasma [K$^+$] may occur *in vitro* associated with marked leukocytosis or thrombocytosis.

Pseudohypokalaemia is less common than pseudohyperkalaemia but can occur due to K^+ uptake into metabolically active cells. If blood with a high leukocyte count is allowed to stand at room temperature for a long period then there will be an intracellular shift of K^+ into the leukocytes. Hypothermia *in vivo* can result in an intracellular shift of K^+ and on rewarming this may result in an overshoot hyperkalaemia.

Summary

K^+ is the major intracellular cation and diffusion of K^+ out of the cell determines the resting membrane potential. Changes in plasma $[K^+]$ primarily affect the electrical activity of the heart. Plasma $[K^+]$ is not a good guide to the total body stores of K^+ which may be depleted despite a normal or raised plasma $[K^+]$. Dietary intake of K^+ is usually more than sufficent to maintain body stores and hypokalaemia is usually caused by prolonged vomiting which restricts intake and causes alkalaemia. The normal kidney can readily excrete excess K^+ and hyperkalaemia is usually found when renal function is limited.

9 Regulation of calcium, magnesium and phosphate balance

The regulation of the three ions Ca^{++}, Mg^{++} and phosphate can be considered as a single topic as the control mechanisms for the three ions are closely related.

The major body stores of Ca^{++}, Mg^{++} and phosphate are within bone and only a tiny fraction is found within extracellular fluid. Under normal conditions the absorption of these ions by the gastrointestinal tract is balanced by renal excretion.

Calcium

Calcium homeostasis

Ninety-nine per cent of Ca^{++} is found in bone and of the remainder almost 1% is within the intracellular compartment and around 0.1% within the extracellular fluid. Although only a tiny fraction of the body store of Ca^{++} is within the extracellular fluid, the plasma $[Ca^{++}]$ is closely controlled. The large store of Ca^{++} in bone is in the form of hydroxyapatite crystals and the $[Ca^{++}]$ in the fluid around the crystals is controlled by means of osteoclast-mediated resorption of bone.

Although only around 1% of the body store of Ca^{++} is found outside bone the Ca^{++} in solution plays a vital role in controlling the activity of excitable tissues. Extracellular $[Ca^{++}]$ influences neuromuscular transmission and cardiac muscle excitability. The normal total plasma $[Ca^{++}]$ is 5 meq/litre (10 mg/decilitre) but it is only the free, ionised Ca^{++} that is physiologically active. Since half of the Ca^{++} in plasma is bound to proteins or other anions the free ionised $[Ca^{++}]$ is around 2.5 meq/litre (5 mg/decilitre). The availability of ionised Ca^{++} is influenced by the presence of other electrolytes; HCO_3^- and phosphate reduce the availability, and H^+ increase the availability.

Changes in the plasma $[Ca^{++}]$ are not always followed by a similar change in the ionised $[Ca^{++}]$ as an increase in plasma albumin concentration will increase total plasma $[Ca^{++}]$ without any change in the ionised $[Ca^{++}]$. A low plasma $[Ca^{++}]$ associated with hypoalbuminaemia is not indicative of hypocalcemia as the physiologically active, ionised $[Ca^{++}]$ may be normal.

Normal $[Ca^{++}]$ intake is around 1 gm per day of which around one third is absorbed across the intestinal mucosa and two thirds lost in the faeces. In order to remain in Ca^{++} balance the renal excretion of Ca^{++} must over a period of time equal the amount absorbed across the intestine. This, however, is not true in the growing child or the pregnant mother where a positive Ca^{++} balance is maintained.

The plasma $[Ca^{++}]$ is controlled by two hormones, parathyroid hormone and vitamin D.

Parathyroid hormone is an 84 amino acid peptide secreted from the parathyroid glands. Hypocalcemia is a potent stimulus for the secretion of parathyroid hormone and hypercalcemia inhibits the secretion of parathyroid hormone as illustrated in Fig. 9.1.

Parathyroid hormone increases plasma $[Ca^{++}]$ by:

1. stimulating bone resorption;
2. increasing renal reabsorption of Ca^{++};
3. stimulating the activation of vitamin D to 1,25-dihydroxycholicalciferol which then increases Ca^{++} absorption by the intestine and stimulates bone resorption.

In order for parathyroid hormone to exert its full effects on bone resorption and Ca^{++} absorption across the intestine there must be an adequate intake of vitamin D. Vitamin D can be taken in the diet as vitamin D (cholecalciferol) and 7- dehydrocholesterol. 7- dehydrocholestrol is converted to (cholecalciferol) in the skin by ultraviolet light. Vitamin D (cholecalciferol) is relatively inactive until it has been hydroxylated first in the liver and then the kidneys to form 1,25- dihydroxycholecalciforol. The active hormone 1,25- dihydroxycholecalciforol circulates in the blood to the target tissues of the intestine and bone as illustrated in Fig. 9.2. 1,25-dihydroxycholecalciferol increases plasma $[Ca^{++}]$ by stimulating Ca^{++} absorption across the intestine and increasing bone resorption.

The renal tubule reabsorbs around 97–98% of the Ca^{++} in the filtrate. Most of the Ca^{++} is reabsorbed passively in proportion to Na^+ and water. Parathyroid hormone stimulate Ca^{++} reabsorption in the distal convoluted tubule and although only 5–10% of the filtered Ca^{++} is reabsorbed by this route it is an important site for hormonal control of Ca^{++} excretion.

The plasma $[Ca^{++}]$ is regulated by parathyroid hormone secretion which controls renal, intestinal and bone mechanisms which restore plasma $[Ca^{++}]$. Parathyroid hormone increases renal reabsorption of Ca^{++} and hypocalcaemia is compensated by hypocalciuria, and hypercalcemia by hypercalciuria.

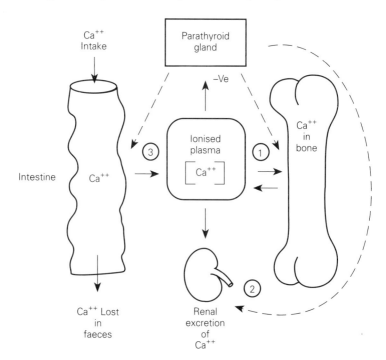

Fig. 9.1   Calcium homeostasis. Ca^{++} intake is balanced by loss of Ca^{++} in the faeces and urine. Only the ionised Ca^{++} in plasma is physiologically active and ionised plasma $[Ca^{++}]$ is regulated by secretion of parathyroid hormone. An increase in plasma $[Ca^{++}]$ inhibits parathyroid hormone secretion. Parathyroid hormone has three main actions as illustrated by the dashed lines (1) to increase bone resorption, (2) to increase the renal reabsorption of Ca^{++}, (3) to increase the absorption of Ca^{++} across the intestine (mediated by 1, 25-dihydroxycholecalciferol as discussed in text). Hypocalcemia is a potent stimulus for parathyroid hormone secretion.

Hypocalcaemia

Hypocalcaemia can be a life-threatening emergency as the increased excitability of the neuromuscular system can lead to tetanic seizures and respiratory arrest. With mild hypocalcaemia there may be parasthesias and hyperreflexia. Chvostek sign may be apparent with facial twitching when the facial nerve is tapped. The Trousseau sign of carpal spasm may also be elicited on occluding the blood flow to the arm with inflation of a sphygmomanometer cuff. Hypocalcaemia predisposes to cardiac arrhythmia and the ECG may exhibit a prolonged Q–T interval.

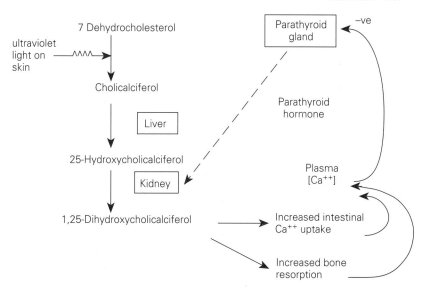

Fig. 9.2 Vitamin D and Calcium homeostasis. Vitamin D can be taken in the diet as cholecalciferol or 7, dehydrocholestrol which is converted to cholecalciferol in the skin on exposure to ultra violet light. Cholecalciferol is hydroxylated in the liver and kidneys to form the hormone 1, 25-dihydroxycholecalciferol. Parathyroid hormone controls the rate limiting hydroxylation of 25-hydroxycholecalciferol in the kidneys. 1, 25-dihydroxycholecalciferol acts to increase plasma [Ca^{++}] by increasing bone resorption and intestinal absorption of Ca^{++}.

Hypocalcaemia is most commonly caused by a reduction in parathyroid hormone secretion and a deficiency of vitamin D and its metabolites. Other causes include unresponsiveness of tissues to parathyroid hormone, increased deposition of Ca^{++} in bone and soft tissues, and chelation of Ca^{++} with citrate following massive blood transfusion.

The most common cause of hypoparathyroidism is damage to the parathyroid glands during thyroidectomy, and plasma [Ca^{++}] should be carefully monitored following surgery of the thyroid gland.

Hypocalcaemia due to vitamin D deficiency may result from prolonged poor absorption of vitamin D associated with malabsorption syndrome. In the West vitamin D deficiency is uncommon as many foods have vitamin D as a supplement.

Pseudohyoparathyroidism is caused by end organ unresponsiveness to parathyroid hormone and this occurs most commonly at the level of the kidney.

Diagnosis of hypocalcaemia

A false hypocalcaemia due to hyperproteinemia should first be eliminated.

The clinical history should look for any indication of thyroid surgery, malabsorption syndrome, and poor dietary intake of vitamin D.

Measurement of plasma phosphate concentration can help in the differential diagnosis. Plasma phosphate will be low if the hypocalcaemia has caused a secondary increase in parathyroid hormone and this may indicate hypocalcaemia due to vitamin D deficiency or calcium malabsorption. Plasma phosphate will be normal to high in cases of hypoparathyroidism or renal failure. Measurement of parathyroid hormone and vitamin D metabolites can give valuable information as parathyroid hormone will be low in hypoparathyroidism and high in cases of vitamin D deficiency and Ca^{++} malabsorption.

Treatment of hypocalcaemia

Hypocalcaemia with any symptoms of increased neuromuscular excitability is treated with intravenous infusion of Ca^{++} in the form of calcium gluconate or other Ca^{++} preparation. Less dangerous situations can be treated with oral calcium preparations and if hypocalcaemia persists these can be supplemented with oral vitamin D preparations. The onset of action of vitamin D is gradual and it has a prolonged effect and caution should be exercised if there is any need to use thiazide diuretics or immobilise the patient as this may result in hypercalcaemia. Thiazide diuretics increase Ca^{++} transport in the renal tubule and reduce urinary Ca^{++} excretion.

Hypercalcaemia

The plasma $[Ca^{++}]$ is determined by three factors; mobilisation of Ca^{++} from bone, renal Ca^{++} absorption, and intestinal absorption of Ca^{++}. Hypercalcaemia could arise from a disturbance in any of these mechanisms but in practice if only one mechanism is disturbed compensation from the others limits any rise in plasma $[Ca^{++}]$. The clinical effects of hypercalcaemia depend on the severity and duration of the disorder. Hypercalcaemia due to excess parathyroid hormone, hyperparathyroidism, can cause peptic ulcer, acute pancreatitis, bone deformity and fractures. Hypercalcaemia can also cause significant psychiatric disturbance with depression, confusion, psychosis and even coma due to central actions on neuronal activity. Hypercalcaemia has little direct effect on neuromuscular activity but can predispose to cardiac arrhythmias and shortening of the Q–T interval. The renal system can be severely affected with hypercalcaemia which can cause a decrease in GFR, renal stone formation, and nephrogenic diabetes insipidus by antagonising the effects of ADH.

The two most common causes of hypercalcaemia are hyperparathyroidism and malignancy, especially with multiple myeloma, breast and lung cancer. Tumours can release humoral factors with parathyroid hormone like activity and cause mobilisation of Ca^{++} from bone. Primary hyperparathyroidism is most commonly due to a parathyroid gland adenoma and excess parathyroid hormone causes bone resorption and increased absorption of Ca^{++} along the intestine and renal tubule.

Diagnosis of hypercalcaemia

Chronic hypercalcaemia indicates primary hyperparathyroidism whereas an acute hypercalcaemia suggests malignancy. A high level of parathyroid hormone in the absence of renal failure suggests primary hyperparathyroidism. A high urinary $[Ca^{++}]$ and low plasma phosphate concentration also support the diagnosis of primary hyperarathyroidism. Hypercalcaemia can be caused by excessive intake of vitamin D especially if used in conjunction with thiazide diuretics which promote renal Ca^{++} reabsorption.

Treatment of hypercalcaemia

Because of the danger of soft tissue calcification and psychiatric disturbance, hypercalcaemia should be treated immediately, even in the absence of any symptoms. Obvious measures include cessation of any current Ca^{++} and vitamin D supplement and mobilisation of patients. Ca^{++} and Na^{+} reabsorption in the renal tubule are closely linked and if Na^{+} excretion can be increased this will cause a fall in plasma $[Ca^{++}]$ by encouraging urinary loss of Ca^{++}. Over 80% of filtered Ca^{++} is reabsorbed in the proximal tubule and loop of Henle and this mechanism of Ca^{++} reabsorption can be diminished by expansion of extracellular fluid volume. Treatment of hypercalcaemia should therefore include expansion of the extracellular fluid volume especially if there is any dehydration due to nephrogenic diabetes insipidus. Diuresis and increased Ca^{++} loss can be maintained by saline infusion or dextrose infusion.

Hypophosphataemia may be present with hyperparathyroidism and oral phosphates are required if the plasma phosphate concentration is below 3 mg/decilitre. Inhibitors of bone resorption have a limited use in hypercalcaemia as they have only a moderate action and toxic side effects.

Phosphorus

Phosphorus like Ca^{++} is mainly found in bone (85%) but unlike Ca^{++} there is up to 14% of body phosphorus found within the intracellular compartment. Phosphorus is found mainly as phosphate (dibasic HPO_4^{2-} and monobasic $H_2PO_4^{-}$). Movement of phosphate between the extracellular and cellular compartments can have a marked effects on plasma phosphate concentration. Phosphate is an important component of DNA, RNA and ATP, and acts as a urinary and intracellular buffer. Only a trace of the total body phosphorus is found in the extracellular compartment and plasma phosphate concentration is around 4 mg/decilitre. The plasma concentration of total phosphate is around 12 mg/decilitre but much of this is organic phosphate. The normal clinical laboratory value given for phosphate is for acid soluble phosphate which us usually around 4 mg/decilitre. Plasma phosphate concentration is not closely controlled when compared with $[Ca^{++}]$ which is regulated in a narrow range by parathyroid hormone. Phosphate concentration fluctuates with a diurnal rhythm and is influenced by arterial PCO_2 and carbohydrate intake.

Phosphate homeostasis

Phosphate homeostasis is determined by a balance between absorption of phosphate across the intestine and renal excretion of phosphate. A normal Western diet contains more than sufficient phosphate, and absorption across the intestine regulates uptake, with over one third of ingested phosphate normally lost in the faeces. Vitamin D has an important role in phosphate homeostasis, as the active metabolite 1,25- dihydroxycholecalciferol enhances intestinal phosphate transport. Parathyroid hormone has little direct action on the intestinal uptake of phosphate but increases phosphate uptake indirectly by promoting the renal formation of 1, 25- dihydroxycholecalciferol.

The metabolism of Ca^{++} and phosphate are closely linked in bone as parathyroid hormone and the active form of vitamin D, 1, 25- dihydroxycholecalciferol cause bone resorption and release of Ca^{++} and phosphate.

The kidneys are the main regulator of plasma phosphate concentration by both direct and indirect mechanisms as shown in Fig. 9.3. The renal threshold for phosphate excretion is very close to the normal plasma concentration of phosphate and any increase in plasma phosphate concentration rapidly leads to urinary excretion of phosphate. In that sense, the kidneys actually regulate plasma phosphate concentration. The capacity of the kidneys to reabsorb phosphate can be influenced by parathyroid hormone and dietary intake of phosphate. Parathyroid hormone decreases phosphate reabsorption at the renal tubule and increases urinary excretion of phosphate. Similarly, a high phosphate diet increases urinary excretion of phosphate by a mechanism which appears to be independent of parathyroid hormone. Hypophosphataemia can increase intestinal uptake of phosphate by stimulating the formation of 1,25 -dihydroxycholecalciferol via the kidneys.

Hypophosphataemia

Chronic hypophosphataemia causes a depletion of body phosphate stores with osteomalacia and myopathy. Hypophosphataemia may also cause non specific psychiatric disorders similar to chronic hypercalcaemia with paraesthesia, confusion and coma.

Three basic mechanisms can cause hypophosphataemia; a reduction in intestinal uptake of phosphate, increased urinary excretion of phosphate and an intracellular shift of phosphate.

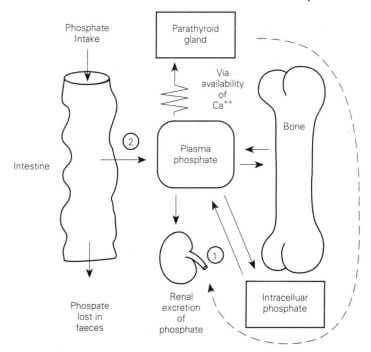

Fig. 9.3 There is no direct hormonal control of plasma phosphate concentration. Changes in plasma phosphate concentration influence the availability of ionised Ca^{++} and this can secondarily affect the secretion of parathyroid hormone which controls the renal excretion of phosphate (1). The uptake of phosphate across the intestine (2) is enhanced by 1, 25-dihydroxycholicalciferol and a fall in plasma phosphate stimulates the formation of this active metabolite of vitamin D by the kidneys. Most of the body phosphate store is within bone and the intracellular compartment, and movement of phosphate in and out of these stores can cause major changes in plasma phosphate concentration.

A reduction in intestinal uptake of phosphate may be the result of malabsorption syndrome as this can result in vitamin D deficiency and a reduction in intestinal uptake of phosphate. With vitamin D deficiency a secondary increase in parathyroid hormone secretion will cause an increased urinary excretion of phosphate.

Increased urinary excretion of phosphate is caused by any primary or secondary increase in the secretion of parathyroid hormone and this can result in hypophosphataemia. The plasma phosphate level rarely falls below 2 mg/decilitre with primary hyperparathyroidism but with secondary hyperparathyroidism due to vitamin D deficiency the reduced intestinal absorption of phosphate can cause more severe hypophosphataemia.

The intracellular store of phosphate is much greater than the phosphate found in extracellular fluid and consequently any intracellular shift of phosphate can cause severe acute hypophosphataemia. The process of glycolysis causes conversion of inorganic phosphate to organic phosphate and the reduction in intracellular inorganic phosphate causes an intracellular shift of phosphate. Administration of carbohydrates such as fructose and glucose stimulate glycolysis and cause hypophosphataemia. Similarly, insulin, glucagon and catecholamines can cause hypophosphataemia by stimulating glycolysis. Hypophosphataemia can also be caused by respiratory alkalosis which stimulates glycolysis and shifts phosphate towards the intracellular compartment. Ingestion of phosphate binding antacids is a common cause of hypophosphataemia but this only rarely causes osteomalacia.

Diagnosis of hypophosphataemia

In general, chronic hypophosphataemia is caused by renal phosphate loss and acute phosphataemia by an intracellular shift of phosphate. Diagnosis of acute hypophosphataemia can be based on plasma phosphate level and a history of carbohydrate administration, respiratory alkalosis, or other factors causing an intracellular shift of phosphate. Measurement of urinary phosphate level can help in the differential diagnosis of chronic hypophosphataemia as a high urinary phosphate level indicates renal wasting and a low level indicates malabsorption and vitamin D deficiency. Measurement of parathyroid hormone helps to confirm primary hyperparathyroidism when hypophosphataemia is associated with hypercalcaemia. Secondary hyperparathyroidism due to vitamin D deficiency is associated with hypocalcemia and hypophosphataemia.

Treatment of hypophosphataemia

In the case of an acute shift of phosphate into cells treatment is not usually necessary as body stores of phosphate are normal and there is no shortage of intracellular organic phosphate such as ATP and 2,3–DPG. Only when there is a long-standing depletion of body phosphate does an acute intracellular shift of phosphate cause intracellular damage.

Intravenous therapy is reserved for severe hypophosphatemia with neuromuscular symptoms. Care should be taken that phosphate infusion does not cause hypocalaemia as an increase in plasma phosphate will reduce the availability of ionised Ca^{++}. Oral phosphate and an increase intake of dairy products which contain high levels of phosphorus can be used to treat modest hypophosphataemia once treatment has been initiated to correct any malabsorption or renal problem.

Hyperphosphataemia

Acute hyperphosphataemia can cause hypocalcemia by reducing the availability of ionised Ca^{++} in plasma. Hypocalcaemia is only a risk with acute hyperphosphataemia as parathyroid hormone secretion restores plasma $[Ca^{++}]$ in chronic hyperphosphataemia. The main complication of chronic hyperphosphataemia is deposition of Ca^{++} in soft tissues such as kidney, heart, lungs, conjunctiva, and skin.

There are three main causes of hyperphosphataemia; (1) a shift of phosphate from the intracellular to the extracellular compartment, (2) an increased intake of phosphate, (3) reduced renal excretion of phosphate.

The large store of phosphate in cells means that any major cell damage which releases cell contents can cause hyperphosophataemia. Red blood cell or muscle cell injury due to trauma, infection, etc. can cause an acute hyperphosphataemia. Similarly, the breakdown of a large number of tumour cells during treatment can cause acute hyperphosphataemia.

Administration of excessive phosphate in the form of antacids or other substances can cause an acute hyperphosphataemia but this is usually only apparent when there is a reduction in the ability of the kidney to excrete phosphate.

A reduction in GFR due to renal failure or hypovolaemia can lead to phosphate retention and hyperphosphataemia. The most common cause of chronic hyperphosphataemia is a reduction in renal phosphate excretion due to hypoparathyroidism or unresponsiveness of the kidney to parathyroid hormone (pseudohypoparathyroidism).

Diagnosis of hyperphosphataemia

An increase in plasma phosphate concentration to over 4.5 mg/decilitre can be defined as hyperphosphataemia. Acute elevation of plasma phosphate concentration may greatly exceed this level without any tissue damage but chronic hyperphosphataemia causes calcium deposition in soft tissues. Symptoms of acute hyperphosphataemia are mainly those of hypocalcaemia with neuromuscular excitability and parasthesias.

Urinary phosphate is elevated in hyperphosphataemia due to excessive phosphate intake and release of phosphate from the cellular compartment but is reduced in cases of renal failure, hypovolaemia and hypoparathyroidism.

Because of the great capacity of the kidney to excrete excess phosphate a reduction in GFR is usually a causative factor in hyperphosphataemia and GFR should be estimated by creatinine clearance or plasma creatinine concentration to assess the degree of any renal involvement.

Treatment of hyperphosphataemia

With normal renal function excess phosphate is readily excreted and the first goal of therapy should be to improve GFR if possible. If hypovolaemia is present then this should be corrected and the subsequent increase in urine output may be sufficient to lower plasma phosphate concentration back towards normal. If GFR is very low due to renal failure then haemodialysis may be necessary in order to lower plasma phosphate concentration.

Treatment of asymptomatic hyperphosphataemia can be achieved by a low phosphate diet and avoidance of dairy products. If necessary phosphorous binding agents such as calcium carbonate can be combined with a low phosphate diet.

Magnesium

Mg^{++} is found mainly in bones and the intracellular compartment. Less than 1% of body stores of Mg^{++} is found in the extracellular compartment. Mg^{++} has similar physiological actions to Ca^{++} as plasma $[Mg^{++}]$ influences neuromuscular excitability. Hypomagnesaemia causes increased neuromuscular excitability and hypermagnesaemia depresses the activity of cardiac and skeletal muscle. Intracellular Mg^{++} is mainly bound to enzymes, protein, nucleic acids and organelles.

Magnesium homeostasis

There is normally more than sufficient Mg^{++} intake in a normal Western diet. Approximately one third of the dietary Mg^{++} is absorbed across the intestine and this intake is balanced by an equal renal excretion of Mg^{++}. The kidneys have a great capacity to excrete excess Mg^{++} and dietary overload is rare if renal function is normal. In contrast to other electrolytes where renal reabsorption occurs primarily at the proximal tubule over half of the filtered load of Mg^{++} is reabsorbed at the loop of Henle. The reabsorption of Mg^{++} is linked to that of Na^+ and loop diuretics cause loss of Mg^{++} in the urine. With a reduction in dietary intake the intestinal absorption of Mg^{++} is increased and renal excretion reduced. In contrast to other electrolytes there does not appear to be any hormonal mechanism regulating the plasma concentration and body stores of Mg^{++}. The plasma $[Mg^{++}]$ is approximately 2 meq/litre (2 mg/decilitre) and this is determined by a balance between intestinal absorption, renal excretion and exchange with bone and the intracellular compartment.

Hypomagnesaemia

The symptoms of hypomagnesaemia are similar to those of hypocalcaemia with increased neuromuscular excitability. Hypomagnesaemia is often associated with hypocalcaemia and hypokalaemia. Hypomagnesaemia may be caused by a decrease in Mg^{++} intake due to starvation, malabsorption or diarrhoea. Increased renal excretion of Mg^{++} due to extracellular volume expansion or the use of loop diuretics can also cause hypomagnesaemia.

Treatment of severe symptomatic hypomagnesaemia requires infusion of magnesium sulphate solution but asymptomatic hypomagnesaemia can be treated with oral magnesium supplement.

Hypermagnesaemia

Hypermagnesaemia depresses neuromuscular transmission by inhibition of acetyl choline release and symptoms include muscle weakness, hyporeflexia, lethargy and nausea. Very severe hypermagnesaemia can cause cardiac arrest.

The most common cause of hypermagnesaemia is a reduction in GFR due to renal failure. Parenteral Mg^{++} is used in the treatment of eclampsia but any hypermagnesaemia associated with infusion of Mg^{++} is usually of short duration if renal function is normal.

Mild asymptomatic hypermagnesaemia in the course of renal failure does not usually require treatment. Ca^{++} antagonises the effects of Mg^{++} on neuromuscular excitability and a slow intravenous injection of calcium gluconate rapidly reverses the neuromuscular and cardiovascular depressant effects of Mg^{++}.

If renal function is normal then expansion of the extracellular fluid volume and administration of loop diuretics both promote renal excretion of Mg^{++}. In the case of chronic renal failure haemodialysis effectively reduces the plasma $[Mg^{++}]$.

Summary

Ca^{++} Mg^{++} and phosphate are found mainly within bone and the intracellular compartment. The extracellular concentration of these ions has a marked effect on the excitability of the neuromuscular system. The homeostasis of the three ions is a balance between intestinal absorption and renal excretion which are regulated by parathyroid homone and the active metabolites of vitamin D.

10   Cardiovascular shock

Cardiovascular shock is caused by a decrease in cardiac output associated with inadequate tissue perfusion.

Since the systemic circulation is a 'circuit', disturbances in peripheral resistance, blood volume and venous return all influence cardiac output. Despite this link between all components of the circuit it is simpler to discuss and explain cardiovascular shock in terms of decreased cardiac output.

Cardiovascular shock may be divided into three general types:

1. hypovolaemic shock;
2. low resistance shock;
3. cardiogenic shock.

Hypovolaemic shock

This is literally described as shock caused by an inadequate blood volume and which may be caused by:

1. loss of blood, haemorrhage;
2. loss of plasma, burns, renal disease;
3. loss of water and solute, sweating, dehydration, diarrhoea.

All of the above cause a decrease in blood volume and if this is only a moderate decrease of 5–15 ml/kg or 350 ml–1 litre of blood volume, then the mean arterial blood pressure will be maintained and subsequent intake of fluid will expand the blood volume back to normal. This is an everyday occurrence with blood donations at blood banks and although it may be several weeks before the red blood cell count returns to normal it is only a few hours before blood volume is restored after fluid intake. The arterial blood pressure, blood volume and blood composition are controlled by several compensatory mechanisms but for ease of discussion these may be divided into *immediate compensatory mechanisms* and *long-term compensatory mechanisms*.

Immediate compensatory mechanisms

The immediate compensatory mechanisms are activated by the arterial barroreceptors which sense a fall in arterial blood pressure. If blood volume is decreased, for example due to blood loss, then venous return to the heart is decreased, this causes a decrease in cardiac output which further causes a fall in arterial blood pressure. The immediate compensatory response occurs over a matter of seconds to minutes and involves tachycardia, venoconstriction, and an increase in total peripheral resistance due to arterial vasoconstriction in selected circulations. These responses are caused by an increased release of noradrenaline from sympathetic nerves supplying the heart, veins and peripheral arterioles.

It is often a source of confusion as to how a fall in blood pressure influences the barroreceptors to cause an increase in sympathetic nervous activity. Here it is important to remember that the barroreceptor input to the medullary sympathetic control is inhibitory and that a rise in arterial blood pressure normally stimulates the barroreceptors and inhibits sympathetic activity. With a fall in arterial blood pressure there is a release of inhibitory activity as the barroreceptor activity declines.

The immediate compensatory responses are illustrated in Fig. 10.1 which is a diagram of the cardiovascular circuit. Peripheral vasoconstriction occurs mainly in skin, gut and renal circulations and this diverts blood towards the vital circulations of the heart, lungs and brain. A cold pale skin, which may also be damp due to sweating related to anxiety rather than thermoregulation, is typical of cardiovascular shock. With severe shock the skin of the lips and nail beds may also be cyanosed due to hypoxia. The peripheral vasoconstriction increases the total peripheral resistance and this will tend to maintain the arterial pressure head required for perfusion of the heart, lungs and brain.

Two thirds of the blood volume is held within the veins and this can be considered as a spare tank of blood which can be mobilised in emergency. Venoconstriction occurs in response to blood loss and this squeezes blood from the veins into the arteries and peripheral circulation. The veins shrink around a decreased blood volume and this helps to maintain venous pressure and venous return to the heart. Because of the large cross-sectional area of the veins and the elliptical cross-sectional shape of the large veins, the venoconstriction does not significantly increase the venous resistance to blood flow. In fact the opposite occurs, as venous return is improved. The maintenance of adequate venous return is probably one of the most important factors in cardiovascular shock because the heart can only pump out what it receives and any fall in venous return results in a similar fall in cardiac output.

The compensatory tachycardia which occurs in response to a fall in arterial blood pressure will increase cardiac output only if venous return is maintained. The tachycardia increases the oxygen consumption of the heart and if the hypovolemia is severe and associated with hypoxia the tachycardia may precipitate heart damage.

The increased sympathetic nervous activity will normally be supplemented by an increased release of adrenaline from the adrenal medulla. Adrenaline similarly causes vasoconstriction in skin, gut and renal circula-

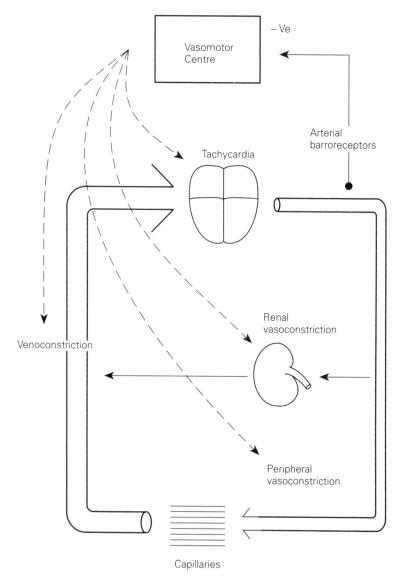

Fig. 10.1   Immediate compensatory mechanisms for hypovolaemia. A fall in arterial blood pressure causes a decrease in arterial barroreceptor activity and decreased inhibition of the vasomotor centre. This results in an increase in sympathetic nervous activity with, tachycardia, venoconstriction and peripheral vasoconstriction.

tions, and also increases blood sugar by promoting glycogenolysis in the liver.

The vasoconstriction in skin, gut and renal circulations maintains the arterial pressure head for the vital organs during the first few minutes and hours of blood loss. This vasoconstriction may be so severe as to almost abolish the blood flow in these organs. Skin, gut and kidney are relatively resistant to hypoxia but their basal metabolic activity will produce lactic acid and other anaerobic metabolites which eventually leak into the systemic circulation. A lactic acidosis is therefore a consequence of the vasoconstriction and this may be accompanied by decreased renal function and sometimes anuria.

Restlessness associated with anxiety and hyperventilation caused by lactic acidosis can be beneficial as both promote venous return by means of the peripheral muscle pump and the respiratory pump.

Although it may not be possible for the patient to immediately take in fluid to restore the blood volume the volume deficit can be made up by a shift of fluid from the interstitial fluid compartment into the blood vascular compartment. Such a movement of fluid is caused by arterial vasoconstriction which reduces the capillary hydrostatic pressure at the arterial end of the capillary. Since the movement of fluid across the capillary is a balance between the outward filtration hydrostatic pressure and the inward reabsorption oncotic pressure of plasma proteins, a reduction in hydrostatic pressure results in net reabsorption of interstitial fluid. Since the volume of interstitial fluid is over three times greater than that of plasma there is a significant reservoir of fluid to compensate for blood loss. This shift of interstitial fluid occurs during the first few hours of peripheral vasoconstriction and helps to maintain the blood volume.

Long-term compensatory mechanisms

The immediate compensatory mechanisms primarily involve the sympathetic vasoconstrictor response which can be initiated in seconds and persist for hours. There is overlap in time with the long-term compensatory mechanisms which involve hormonal responses that can be initiated in the first few hours but which may persist for days. The hormones involved in the long-term compensatory responses are ADH secreted from the posterior pituitary, aldosterone from the adrenal cortex, and erythropoietin from the kidney. The kidney plays a central role in the long-term compensatory response and any renal damage or limitation of function due to prolonged vasoconstriction will obviously limit the capacity to restore blood volume. The factors influencing aldosterone and ADH secretion are illustrated in Fig. 10.2. A decrease in blood volume causes decreases in venous return, cardiac output, arterial blood pressure and renal perfusion. The decrease in renal perfusion causes the release of renin from the kidney which in turn acts on angiotensinogen in the blood to form angiotensin. Angiotensin stimulates the release of aldosterone from the adrenal cortex which in turn stimulates Na^+ reabsorption by the renal tubule.

Increased Na^+ retention alone cannot increase blood volume as the increased body solute must be accompanied by an increased water retention. Water balance is regulated by detecting changes in plasma osmolarity and as soon as Na^+ retention causes an increase in plasma osmolarity this will stimulate the hypothalamic osmoreceptors to cause increased secretion of ADH. Hence as plasma aldosterone levels rise so does plasma ADH.

There are two other mechanisms shown in Fig. 10.2 which also influence ADH release. The filling of the right atrium stimulates atrial

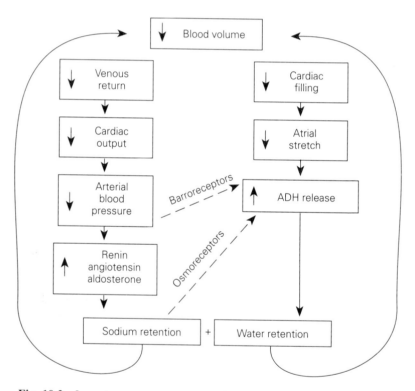

Fig. 10.2 Long term compensatory mechanisms for hypovolaemia. A fall in blood volume causes a decrease in venous return and cardiac filling which eventually lead to an increase in the secretion of aldosterone and antidiuretic hormone (ADH). The main mechanism triggering aldosterone release is increased renin secretion caused by a fall in renal perfusion. ADH release is increased by three mechanisms; increased plasma osmolarity, decreased atrial filling and a fall in arterial blood pressure. The retention of sodium and water causes a return towards normal blood volume.

stretch receptors, and increases in arterial blood pressure stimulate barroreceptors. Both of these stimuli normally inhibit ADH release via sensory nerves in the IX and X cranial nerves. Therefore when blood volume decreases, the decreased filling of the right artium and the decreased arterial blood pressure cause a release from these inhibitory sensory inputs and ADH secretion is increased.

Water can only be retained after ingestion, and in the conscious patient fluid intake is stimulated by the sensation of thirst caused by angiotensin. In the unconscious patient blood volume will not be restored until intravenous fluid replacement therapy is started.

If loss of whole blood is the cause of hypovolaemia then the above mechanisms will restore blood pressure and blood volume, but the haematocrit or packed cell volume will be below normal. Restoration of circulating red cell mass is brought about by increased secretions of the hormone erythropoietin from the kidney in response to renal hypoxia. Lost plasma proteins must also be replaced but the mechanisms stimulating increased production from the liver are unknown.

Irreversible shock

If the hypovolaemia is not life threatening and fluid therapy is initiated within the first few hours then blood volume and blood pressure can be returned within the normal range. However if a patient in hypovolaemic shock is left untreated over many hours then the compensatory mechanisms which maintain perfusion of the vital organs may eventually cause tissue damage. Subsequent fluid therapy then fails to restore blood volume as the fluids escape into the interstitial fluid space. Blood volume and pressure can be transiently restored with fluid therapy but the recovery is short lived and the prognosis is poor.

The mechanism for the tissue damage associated with irreversible shock is prolonged vasoconstriction in skin, gut and renal circulations which cause tissue hypoxia and the accumulation of acid metabolites. Over a period of hours tissue hypoxia and acidaemia causes damage to the capillaries and arterioles. The capillary cells become separated causing a great increase in capillary permeability and the arteriole smooth muscle suffers damage which causes it to relax with subsequent arteriolar vasodilation. The arteriole vasodilation and increased capillary permeability cause a movement of fluid and solute from the vascular space into interstitial fluid. Subsequent transfusions of fluids only cause a transient recovery as fluids are eventually lost into the interstitial space.

Prolonged renal vasoconstriction may cause renal failure which will further complicate the condition with increased loss of solute and water via the damaged kidneys.

The obvious way to prevent tissue damage is to restore blood volume as quickly as possible with intravenous fluid therapy being the treatment of choice. However, several centres have also recommended reversal of the sympathetic arteriolar vasoconstriction by use of alpha antagonists such as phentolamine or beta stimulants such as isoprenaline. The reasoning behind the use of alpha antagonists is that rapid reversal of the peripheral vasoconstriction prevents tissue damage due to hypoxia.

Low resistance shock

Low resistance shock is caused by a decrease in total peripheral resistance due to arteriolar vasodilation. The heart normally pumps blood through the parallel resistances of the peripheral circulations with most of the arterioles in a constricted condition. If a majority of the arterioles were to dilate simultaneously then the blood pressure would fall and blood would pool in the peripheral circulation. Low resistance shock may be classified as:

1.   vaso-vagal syncope;
2.   anaphylactic shock;
3.   septic shock.

Vasovagal syncope

Vasovagal syncope or faint usually occurs in response to fear, pain or stress. There is considerable variation between individuals in their response to stress as some subjects may faint at the sight of a syringe and needle whereas others may only faint with extreme pain.

Vasovagal syncope as the name implies involves arteriolar vasodilation and vagal bradycardia. The vasodilation is believed to occur in arteriovenous shunts in skeletal muscle under the influence of sympathetic cholinergic vasodilator nerves. Vasodilation in the skeletal muscle circulation causes a rapid fall in arterial blood pressure. The fall in arterial blood pressure is further amplified by a vagal bradycardia which reduces cardiac output. The sudden fall in arterial blood pressure reduces blood flow to the cerebral circulation and cerebral hypoxia causes loss of consciousness. The vasovagal syncope is usually short lived and recovery occurs spontaneously in a matter of minutes. Allowing the patient to lie down on the floor rather than sit in a chair aids recovery by promoting venous return to the heart. The tilt couches found in most dentist surgeries not only aid the posture of the dentist but also aid recovery from vasovagal syncope.

Anaphylactic shock

Atopic patients who are hypersensitive to drugs such as penicillin or individuals hypersensitive to insect bites or other allergens are likely to suffer from anaphylactic shock. Shock is caused by a massive release of histamine and other mediators from basophil leukocytes throughout the body. Exposure of the individual to the relevant allergen triggers the anaphylactic shock.

Histamine causes widespread arteriolar vasodilation, venoconstriction, increased capillary permeability and bronchoconstriction. These actions cause a fall in arterial blood pressure, movement of vascular fluid into the interstitial space and hypoxia. In sensitive individuals anaphylactic shock can develop after only a few minutes exposure to the allergen, and rapid treatment is necessary to prevent brain damage or death.

Adrenaline given intravenously is the first line of treatment as the vaso-constriction and tachycardia caused by adrenaline raise arterial blood pressure. Adrenaline may also inhibit histamine release from basophils. Antihistamines are a second line of treatment as they antagonise the actions of histamine and corticosteroids may be used to dampen down the anaphylactic response to allergen.

Septic shock

Septic shock is caused by overwhelming bacterial infection and the production of bacterial toxins. Earlier classifications attempted to describe the shock according to the nature of the infecting organism but this has proved useless and now septic shock is usually classified as either 'early' or 'late' phases.

In the early phase of septic shock the patient usually appears to be pink and well perfused. Fever is often present with cutaneous vasodilation. The early phase has also been described as 'hyperdynamic' as cardiac output may be increased above normal with tachycardia. Despite the increased cardiac output blood pressure is usually below normal because of a decrease in total peripheral resistance due to the vasodilator effects of bacterial toxins. Even with circulating bacterial toxins some vascular beds may still be constricted such as gut and kidney in response to the low arterial blood pressure. In this early phase of septic shock so long as the blood volume is maintained the increased cardiac outputs can sustain the arterial blood pressure in the face of a very low total peripheral resistance.

In the 'late' phase or hypodynamic phase increased vascular permeability causes a shift of vascular fluid to the interstitial space. Protein, water and solutes extravasate and widespread coagulation may be triggered by bacterial toxins and complement activation. In contrast to the vasodilation of the 'early' phase, the 'late' phase is associated with cutaneous vasoconstriction and the skin is cold and pale. Cardiac output falls as a decrease in blood volume causes decreased venous return. Arterial blood pressure is low and the patient is now in a critical condition dependent on continuous intravenous infusion of fluid to replace losses into the interstitial space.

Treatment of septic shock involves maintenance of blood volume with intravenous fluids, antibiotics and any necessary surgical interventions to drain pus or clean sites of infection.

Cardiogenic Shock

Cardiogenic shock is associated with acute myocardial infarction rather than heart failure due to chronic heart disease. Damage to the heart muscle caused by ischaemia affects cardiac performance and causes a decrease in cardiac output. The decrease in cardiac output causes a fall in arterial blood pressure which triggers an increase in sympathetic activity by the barroreceptor reflex. The sympathetic response is similar to that associated with hypovolaemia with arterial vasoconstriction in skin, gut and kidney accompanied by venoconstriction. Tachycardia often accompanies the peripheral vasoconstriction but in the case of cardiogenic shock this may lead to further ischaemic damage by increasing the oxygen requirements of the heart. The ischaemic damage to heart muscle may itself trigger autonomic reflexes by stimulation of vagal sensory fibres and this may sometimes result in a bradycardia rather than tachycardia. Thus the cardiac response is complicated by the location and the severity of the ischaemic damage.

The peripheral vasoconstriction is part of the immediate compensatory mechanism described above and it will tend to restore arterial blood pressure back to normal.

Despite the fact that there has been no actual decrease in blood volume effective circulating volume is decreased and the long-term compensatory mechanisms involving aldosterone and ADH will be activated as shown in Fig. 10.2. Water and solute retention cause an expansion of blood volume above normal and this is beneficial as it causes increased cardiac filling with an increased end diastolic volume.

Heart muscle exhibits a length tension relationship similar to skeletal muscle and within limits stretching increases the performance of the muscle, and the tension achieved on contraction is greater. The effects of an increase in end diastolic volume on cardiac performance in a healthy and a damaged heart are illustrated in Fig. 10.3. In the case of a damaged heart normal cardiac performance can only be achieved at an increased end diastolic volume. The price the patient pays for this compensated condition is peripheral oedema and a continuous threat of pulmonary oedema. Obviously, in a compensated condition with increased blood volume the use of diuretics could rapidly decrease blood volume and precipitate heart failure and shock. Therefore diuretics should only be used if a life-threatening pulmonary oedema occurs.

Treatment of cardiogenic shock depends on the nature of the cardiac pathology. Treatment of heart failure may involve the use of digitalis which has a positive isotropic action on the heart and increases cardiac output. However if the cardiac failure is due to myocardial infarct then the heart needs to be protected from any increase in work load and in the acute condition vasodilator drugs may reduce the workload and also improve coronary blood flow.

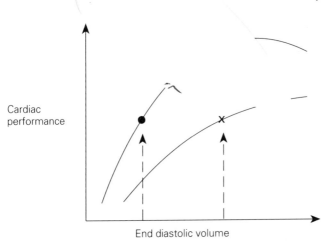

Cardiac
performance

End diastolic volume

Fig. 10.3 Cardiac compensation in heart failure. Cardiac muscle exhibits a length tension relationship similar to skeletal muscle. As resting length (end diastolic volume) increases so the tension achieved on contraction increases. Therefore an increase in blood volume causes increased cardiac filling and an increase in cardiac output. In the case of a damaged heart a normal cardiac performance can only be achieved at an increased end distolic volume. (●) normal condition of heart, (X) damaged heart.

Summary

Cardiovascular shock is caused by a decrease in cardiac output which may be due to blood loss, peripheral vasodilation and cardiac failiure. The compensatory response which maintains arterial blood pressure and the perfusion of the heart, brain and lungs may be divided into immediate and long-term compensatory mechanisms. The immediate response is peripheral vasoconstriction followed by long-term hormonal responses which cause retention of Na+ and water. Treatment of cardiovascular shock aims at restoring the effective circulating volume by improving cardiac output and the perfusion of the peripheral circulation.

Index